# *What others are saying about this book:*

"Everyone has the potential to heal. It is built into us but modern medicine tends to focus on the result and not the cause. **Irene's book can be your life coach and guide you to healing your life and body.** Empower yourself and show up for practice by reading her book and its wisdom."

— Bernie Siegel, MD

*Author of "A Book of Miracles and The Art of Healing" Pediatric surgeon, Author of 12 books on health and healing, a world famous speaker on patient and caregiver issues who is recognized as one of the Top 20 Spiritually Influential Living People on the Planet by the Watkins Review of London, England*

"As a journalist, author, three-time cancer survivor and global patient advocate, I've been on a mission to inspire and inform people about their health choices and help them take charge of their own health care. This book shares that philosophy. **Irene clearly recognizes the power of embracing whatever works best for us from both conventional and integrative medicine.**"

— Jamie Reno

*Author of "Hope Begins In The Dark" and "Snowman on the Pitcher's Mound", award-winning investigative reporter, global patient advocate and three-time cancer survivor*

"The reason **this book is a must-read** is because it guides you through the natural substances. For every drug, with its nasty side effects, there's a natural substance that will do the job better — without the negative effects."

— Burton Goldberg

*Publisher, producer, and author of 18 books on alternative health*

"**This book is an inspiring guide and a powerful tool** for everybody looking not only to heal, but also to be in charge of their healthcare choices."

— Kenneth R. Blanchard, MD, PH.D.

*Author of "What Your Doctor May Not Tell You About Hypothyroidism: A Simple Plan for Extraordinary Results, and "The Functional Approach to Hypothyroidism: Bridging Traditional and Alternative Treatment Approaches for Total Patient Wellness"*

"**This book inspires you to take the initiative** to care for your mind, body and spirit in effective holistic ways. It shows the power of your own determination, drive, and desire to heal yourself - and that with devoted attention you too can do it. **This book makes you want to get up right now and focus every ounce of your effort on living a healthy, clean, positive lifestyle** to infuse every cell in your body with self-care and healing."

— Lisa Fraley, JD,
*Attorney, Legal Coach + Holistic Health Coach*

"What a **powerful resource for health practitioners!** Each of the stories in this book can be used as a great example and as powerful motivation for our clients and patients. This book serves as an important reminder that our bodies have an innate ability to heal and thrive. It is up to us to make the decision to become educated patients and support our health."

— Yuliya Tsitova
*Integrative Nutrition Health Coach, Women's Health and Hormone Cure Coach, "YT Wellness" Founder*

"This book offers a **great collection of insight and advice** that could be of the enormous help to everyone looking for the ways to get and stay healthy and live vibrant life"

— Suzanne Gilad
*Health and Life-Style Coach, NutraMetrix Consultant, Author, Broadway producer*

"The Power of the Educated Patient **provides you with map for your road to recovery** by showing you how others have healed themselves and how you can too!"

— Marie Ann Mosher,
*Author of the Amazon #1 bestseller "Beyond Food", Holistic Health Practitioner*

"As a parent who lived through their child's illness **I wish we had the book like that** back then."

— Debbie Casey

# *Your FREE Bonus Gift*

As a small token of appreciation for buying this book, I'd like to present you with "The Bottom-Line of Identifying Your Best HealthCare" quiz that will help you determine how educated and empowered you are as a patient.

This **FREE quiz** will help you to:
- Discover the **top 3 crucial requirements for healing and vibrant health** shared by every single conqueror of their disease.
- Uncover the **#1 false belief most people have** when they suffer with poor health.
- Learn the fundamental **difference between Conventional** and Integrative approaches.
- Find out **3 major ways** the **conventional office experience** is different from the **unconventional** one.
- Figure out **5 pieces of a puzzle**, that if put together give you the clear picture of the way to **true healing and vibrant health**!

You can download your free gift here:
**www.IreneHealthAndWellnessEducator.com**
**www.ThePowerOfTheEducatedPatient.com**

*Inspiring, Educating and Empowering You as a Patient*

# The Power of the
# Educated Patient

PROVEN STRATEGIES FOR
**RECLAIMING YOUR HEALTH**
AND **WELL-BEING** THAT
YOU WON'T FIND IN A
CONVENTIONAL MEDICAL OFFICE

## IRENE DRABKIN

THE SECRETS TO HOW SAVVY PATIENTS OVER CAME THEIR DISEASES
THROUGH INTEGRATIVE MEDICINE, NATURAL THERAPIES, LIFESTYLE
MODIFICATIONS, AND HEALING FOODS

WHAT CURED THEM, WHY IT WORKS, HOW IT CAN WORK FOR YOU!

THE POWER OF THE EDUCATED PATIENT
Copyright 2015 Irene Drabkin

www.ThePowerOfTheEducatedPatient.com
www.IreneHealthAndWellnessEducator.com

Because of the dynamic nature of the Internet, any web addresses or links contained in this book may have changed since publication and may no longer be valid.

The information provided in this book is for informational purposes only and is not intended as a substitute for advice from the qualified health care professional. This is a reference guide to help readers reach their health goals by helping them devise and implement positive, sustainable lifestyle changes. This guide is not to be relied upon as medical advice and it is not designed to diagnose, prevent, treat or cure any medical disease or condition. If the reader is under the care of a health care professional or currently uses prescription medications, the reader should discuss any dietary changes or potential dietary supplements use with his or her doctor, and should not discontinue any prescription medications without first consulting his or her doctor.

For more information, contact Irene Drabkin at ThePowerOfTheEducatedPatient@gmail.com visit www.ThePowerOfTheEducatedPatient.com

**ISBN-13: 978-1517570736**
**ISBN-10: 1517570735**
**LCCN: 2015916261**

# Table of Contents

## Proven Strategies for Reclaiming Your Health and Well-Being

### Part I: Food Intolerances and Sensitivities

### Part II: Autoimmune Disorders

## Part IX: Environmental Diseases

## Part X: Organ Transplant/Transplant Living

## Part XI: Unknown/Undiagnosed Mystery Disorders

# *Dedication*

*... this could be a book on its own ...*

To the fallen victims of the conventional sick-care system — the careless moneymaking machine it has become.

To the pioneers of Integrative Medicine — the brightest and courageous MDs who are the true healers and superheroes we've always believed doctors are.

To my husband, a highly educated MD, whose scientific background spiced up with a pinch of healthy skepticism was a powerful motivator for me to investigate alternatives to our sick-care system and, consequently, become an actual doctor in our family.

To my beautiful children, Adele and Anthony, who inspire and teach me every day with their genuine desire to understand 'why' and 'how' with absolute openness to unforeseen answers and new ways.

To my parents for their unconditional love and acceptance, for being the best grandparents ever, which allowed me the space in my life to work on this book.

To Ingrid and David for always believing in me and teaching me how to fly when I could barely walk.

To incredible Pnina and Irving; very special Betty and Nevile; exceptional Dena and Martin; loving Sveta and Boris; the late, big-hearted Ian and Mildred Karten; admirable Debra and Margo; the late, magnificent Valerie; inspiring David; cheerful Joyce; and the bravest 35 English Jewish Ladies - for taking me into your hearts and homes when the East/West borders kept my own family thousands of miles away.

**"Our bodies are our gardens –
our wills are our gardeners."**

**~William Shakespeare**

"Integrative medicine is the judicious application of both conventional and evidence-based natural therapies."

— Andrew Weil, MD

"Mind-body medicine should not be an 'alternative,' nor should complementary and integrative medicine be something doctors are not exposed to during their training."

— Bernie Siegel, MD

"Most allopathic doctors think practitioners of alternative medicine are all quacks. They're not. Often they're sharp people who think differently about disease."

— Dr. Mehmet Oz, MD

"Functional medicine is about causes, not symptoms. It is getting to the root of the problem."

— Mark Hyman, MD

"By using the best of both worlds — conventional medicine and alternative medicine — you can have your best opportunity for a healthy outcome."

— Burton Goldberg, health advocate, author, publisher, producer

"Of course, modern medicine has its place and serves an invaluable function when it comes to major trauma and emergency situations. But for most diseases... there are many alternative therapies (including simple dietary changes) that can be *more effective* than conventional medical treatments — not to mention more economical, less harmful and less invasive."

— Dr. Joseph Mercola

# *Acknowledgements*

I'm deeply grateful to all the people who took time from their busy lives to share their health journeys with me: **Andrea Nakayama, Arlene Figueroa, Barbara Searles, Debbie and Kaitlyn Casey, Donna Trapp Grimm, Dr. Karen Moriarty, Dr. Jackie Campisi and Greg Culver, Ellen Allard, Gracelyn Guyol, Janet Verney, Jarod Jacobs, Laura Brown, Nishma Shah, Pamela Schmidlin, Phyllis Traver, Rachael Coburn, Shayna Mahoney, Suzanne Foglio, Tina Marian, TJ Carbone.**

Every single person I talked to provided way more than their stories and healing strategies. They gifted me with a clear vision and courageous determination that, hopefully, I was able to pass on to our readers.

I particularly want to thank **Joshua Rosenthal**, the founder of the school for Integrative Nutrition and one of the most remarkable visionaries and leaders that I know.

Dear Joshua, if not for you, I wouldn't be where I am today. This book certainty wouldn't exist, and its healing stories would have remained hidden from the many people who desperately seek answerers and possibilities. *I know, you know that, but I wanted you to know that I know that!*

**Lindsey Smith** for all of your support, encouragement and for being a great example of what's possible.

**Debbi and Julian Sanzo-Davis** - the founders of the *New Self-Health Movement*, and the most remarkable, generous, genuine and humble human beings I know. Thank you for building a healing community of people where everyone is predestined to grow and shine.

**Chris Simpson**, my amazing editor, not only for enhancing my drawings with beautiful colors but also for providing a gentle guidance that encouraged and empowered me to finish my mission and bring these precious stories out to the world.

**Yuliya Tsitova** and **Daron Migirdeyan** for your invaluable cheer and continuous support.

**Laura Schiff Jack** — for being very generous with your amazing gift of creativity.

**Alina Bas** — for sharing your beautiful mind and brainstorming with me.

**Yelena Spivak** – one of the smartest women I know, for seeing further than many and gladly sharing your vision and wisdom.

**Dr. Peter Duncan** — for your confidence in me, when almost 25 years ago you gave me the chance not only to study at one of the most prestigious universities in London, but also provided me with motivation to prove you right and, consequently, be where I am today.

**Martin Hitchcock** — my first British English writing teacher for showing me both: how writing is done skillfully and how it can be fun.

**Kitsie Henchman-Sallet** — my first American English teacher — for helping me make my Brandeis experience both a smooth sail and a great success.

# *Preface*

## *Why You Need to Be an Educated and Empowered Patient*

> *"Without action to reverse current trends, the health of Americans will probably continue to fall behind that of people in other high-income countries. The tragedy is not that the United States is losing a contest with other countries but that Americans are dying and suffering from illness and injury at rates that are demonstrably unnecessary."*
> — Institute of Medicine, 2013 Report

Our country is one of the wealthiest countries in the world, but it is far from the healthiest. Despite the fact that the American health-care system is one of the most expensive among all developed countries, it was ranked 37th worldwide by the World Health Organization in 2000.

Furthermore, statistics from the Institute of Medicine show that our healthcare is failing us. When compared with our peer countries, we are far worse in a number of health areas, including:

- Infant mortality
- Heart disease
- Drug-related deaths
- Obesity and diabetes
- Injuries and homicides
- HIV and AIDS
- Chronic lung disease
- Disability

I share these facts with you not to scare you, but to emphasize the importance of getting and staying in charge of your healthcare through becoming an educated and empowered patient.

We've been taught to trust our doctors, and we believe they're experts at keeping us in our best health. However, the truth of the matter is that most American medical schools train their students to treat the *symptoms* of disease and not the root cause, not search for the ways to prevent it! Most schools don't offer courses in nutrition and prevention.

I'll never forget how, during one of the holistic health conferences I attended, Dr. Oz was asked what was the most surprising or shocking thing about health and nutrition he discovered throughout *all* his experience as a doctor, and he immediately said: "The most shocking thing about nutrition and health I've discovered as a doctor is that we don't learn about nutrition in medical school. At all."

Thankfully today our "disease management" system is beginning to evolve and is becoming the health-care system we deserve. There is a growing number of integrative health practitioners who are *focused on the root causes of disease rather than symptom relief* and providing health care based on good nutrition and lifestyle.

I am truly honored to be on the forefront of this health movement and to share with you the wisdom and strategies of 20 health experts who started their professional paths with having to overcome their own health challenges.

Learn from this information-packed reference book and implement new ways to create better health and more joy and happiness in your life.

Your best, most vibrant life is waiting for you!

# *Introduction*

*"We need to learn from people who recover and people who stay healthy ...
If you are ill or facing adversity, you can begin to heal yourself by following the
paths others have followed."*
— *Bernie Siegel, M.D.*

Here it is! A reference guide with inspiring stories from people who healed themselves or their loved ones with the help of functional medicine, natural therapies, lifestyle modifications, and healing foods.

I hope this book will help change common conceptions about what healing IS and what it is NOT.

*Proven Strategies for Reclaiming Your Health and Well-Being* demonstrates that true healing is Not about taking a prescription drug to alleviate symptoms. True healing is about getting to the root of a problem and finding a way to solve it and, as a result, cure.

After being unable to find solution within the conventional medical system — one that has transformed us into a drug-dependent nation, where nearly 70 percent of all Americans take at least one prescription drug for a chronic or medical condition — our storytellers embarked on their own health journeys and discovered alternative healing strategies that allowed them to heal.

## The Story Behind the Story:
## the Inspiration Behind This Book

*"As soon as healing takes place, go out and heal somebody else."*
— *Maya Angelou*

I met Shayna a few years ago at the conference for holistic practitioners and asked her what made her choose this career. She told me the story about her father becoming disabled from taking statin drugs and how that forced her to search for help. Eventually, she was able to get him from disability and literally save his life by finding the ways to cure him through the right diet and alternative therapies.

xix

This was the beginning of her holistic journey.

When Shayna was describing the symptoms her father had, I realized that my father had similar symptoms and that he was taking the same drug. After learning about the potential dangers of this drug (officially called "side effects"), I did my own research. I wasn't equipped with enough knowledge to take my father off that drug. In most cases taking a radical action should be done only under the close supervision of a qualified health professional (like an integrative physician). However, I added vital supplementation to my father's medical regiment and that alleviated his major symptoms and saved him from getting worse and, possibly, getting disabled. That is how Shayna's sharing her story about healing her father helped me help my father.

At the time I thought: what if more people can learn this story and it could possibly help them or their loved ones?

Then I realized that I could serve as a messenger and share this and many other healing stories with you.

This is how the idea for the book was born.

## *An Educated Patient Is an Empowered Patient!*

*"The work of the doctor will, in the future, be ever more that of an educator, and ever less that of a man who treats ailments."*
*— Lord Horder*

Regrettably, prescribing a massive number of pharmaceutical drugs has become today's new 'norm.' The truth is, oftentimes it is not making the patient better, but someone else better off. By educating ourselves we can avoid falling into this trap. An educated patient is an empowered patient! This is what I preach and teach.

It is also crucial to remember the concept of bio individuality: no two people are the same, which means that everyone requires a different and unique approach depending on their individual needs.

The stories shared in this book may help you find the healing strategy and approach that is right for you. These stories may point you in the right direction, so you start on your road of recovery and reaching your best vibrant health. Or maybe you simply find hope and encouragement while being inspired by these stories. This is how we become educated empowered patients! This is how we find true healing!

# *What This Book Will Do for You*

*"Every patient carries her or his own doctor inside."*
— *Albert Schweitzer*

If you are looking for a solution to your health challenge and ready for a change, the stories in this book will:

**Educate and Empower You**
Every person I interviewed for this book sought help from conventional and unconventional medical establishments, and each system delivered dramatically different experiences.

Typically **only integrative doctors or practitioners** provided my interviewees with the
- TIME to explain what they felt was wrong
- ATTENTION that made them feel like they were being listened to and HEARD
- TEAM approach as the practitioner worked alongside WITH them

**Save You Time**
No more wasted precious moments looking in the wrong places for the wrong treatments.

**Guide You**
Many of the people had to search for years for a proper diagnosis. And one can't get the right treatment if they don't know what they are treating. That's why each story in the book is followed by a list of symptoms and general information about the condition, so you may recognize the condition you or someone you know is suffering from.

**Surprise You**
Initially, many people sincerely believed that the pain or discomfort they were experiencing was NORMAL. It was their destiny to suffer and nothing could make them feel better except taking a drug for short- term relief.

**Inspire You!**
Learning how others heal themselves significantly boosts your confidence to start your own journey towards recovery!

# *How to Use This Book*

*"In order to effectively battle illness, we must get in touch with our inner selves and work toward the goal of survival by using everything available to us, seen and unseen."*
— *Bernie Siegel, MD*

Each story covers five important steps to getting well. While the illnesses and the healing approaches vary, the principals and strategies apply to us all.

## 1. Disease

Each chapter contains a story of healing a particular disease or complaint.

## 2. Disease → **Symptoms & Triggers**

You can see how the disease had developed, as well as the triggers and the symptoms it caused.

*Astonishingly, a vast number of people are not aware of what exactly they suffer from. However, by learning and comparing the symptoms one can recognize the condition.*

## 3. Disease → Symptoms & Triggers → **Healing Strategy**

Each story takes us on the journey of discovering what works and what doesn't and what is the best strategy that you may decide to implement if you or someone you care for is suffering from the same or similar condition.

## 4. Disease → Symptoms & Triggers → Healing Strategy → **Bio individuality**

Every story is a true revelation of someone's pain, struggle, determination and eventual healing.

These forerunners opened up their *lives* so that you can avoid the mistakes they made on their journeys and learn what worked for them, and why and how it can work for you so that you heal faster while avoiding unnecessary repercussions.

That said, we are all different. Each person has his or her unique genetics and life conditions. Thus, while these tips and strategies may help to heal one person, they may be mainly eye-opening for another, and that will lead them to new possibilities. I suggest you both be open- minded and use your own judgment.

For instance, I never recommend drastic action such as getting off your current drugs without medical supervision.

In most cases you should consult an Integrative Physician or Naturopathic Doctor. These doctors are healers who will guide you through the conventional medical system, away from excessive medication.

These physicians take the time to look at the root of the problem instead of simply prescribing a drug to alleviate symptoms.

However, I do recommend trying new lifestyle strategies, a healing diet, and natural therapies that will make you feel better without interrupting what you've already been doing.

**5. Disease $\rightarrow$ Symptoms&Triggers $\rightarrow$ Healing Strategy $\rightarrow$ Bio individuality**

When you know exactly what you are suffering from, what triggers the symptoms, and what can be done to alleviate these symptoms — you are in a good starting place.

When you add your uniqueness and bio-individuality into the mix and get specifically what works for you and your body — you are on the pathway to true healing!

Compare treatments, symptoms, and experiences with people like you and take control of your health.

By building a toolbox with the strategies from real-life experiences, you will reduce the uncertainty about your current health, enhance the dialogue between you and your doctor, create valuable opportunities for better care, and improve your healthcare choices.

*Proven Strategies for Reclaiming
Your Health and Well-Being*


*Part I*

*Food Intolerances and Sensitivities*

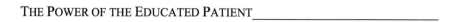

# *My Story (the Beginning)*

*"Life is a succession of lessons which must be lived to be understood."*
— Helen Keller

Last year, our four-year-old son, Anthony, told us he didn't want to grow anymore. We were stunned. Like most children, until that day he couldn't wait to grow up, to be as big and strong as his father. When I asked Anthony why, he said he didn't want his tummy to hurt. The simple explanation he gave was mind-blowing to me. And it made me realize something about human nature that would significantly change the course of my and my family's life.

At that time, Anthony's six-year old sister, Adele, was suffering from severe stomach pain. Anthony assumed this was normal for a child at age six. And he reasoned that when he turned six he'd also get that same, agonizing pain.

Sound familiar? When you think about it, this is what happens to adults, too, and we formulate similar assumptions. As we grow older, we often assume that once we reach a certain age, we're destined to feel "age appropriate." We just accept that we will get certain illnesses, be less energetic, and experience pain. If you're like a lot of people, you consider this to be normal.

Many people I've interviewed for this book shared that, initially, they believed the symptoms they were suffering from were simply a normal part of life. Feeling chronically sick, tired, depressed, and lacking the zest for life they once enjoyed was chalked up to being an unavoidable reality. And I confess that I used to think this way, too.

For the people I interviewed and for me, finding the right doctor, reading the right book, or discovering the right healthcare approach made all the difference in addressing the root causes of illness and imbalance in the body. As a result, alleviating symptoms so the body can heal itself.

Now I want to help you find an effective strategy of using lifestyle changes to overcome your health challenges and reach your ultimate health goals.

Let me start with the story of how I healed Adele and, as a result, got her younger brother, Anthony, excited about growing up again.

# 1
# *A Simple Solution for My Daughter's Terrible Stomach Pain*

*"Something you're eating may be killing you, and you probably don't even know it! The modern wheat is not the wheat your great-grandmother used to bake her bread. It is FrankenWheat — a scientifically engineered food product developed in the last 50 years."*
*— Mark Hyman, MD*

Adele had always been a happy child.

She loved dancing, playing piano, exploring the outdoors, playing with dolls, watching cartoons, and leading the carefree life that only a six-year-old can. But that all changed when she began first grade.

At the beginning of her school year, she started complaining of mild stomach discomfort. Before too long, her symptoms became much worse and terribly worrisome for me. Intense stomach pain, nausea, and bouts of undigested stool plagued my sweet girl on a daily basis.

Because of these debilitating symptoms, Adele soon became fearful of going to school and dreaded the thought of participating in any of the after-school activities she used to love. Fearful of sudden stomach pain, she didn't want to leave the house. When I would drop her off at school in the morning, her eyes would well up with tears as she pleaded with me to not make her go.

In a matter of weeks, my once-happy, joyful first-grader morphed into a scared, socially disabled, depressed child. Our life as a family had become a near constant nightmare filled with worry and angst as we were always waiting for Adele's sickness to strike again. Watching this happen to my little girl and our family, I was heartbroken. I desperately wanted to understand what happened.

Our pediatrician diagnosed Adele with intense heartburn (GERD), which I already figured out at that point. Next, we gave her all of the tests that conventional medicine could offer. She tested negative for celiac disease and gluten intolerance, both common causes of heartburn. To alleviate her symptoms, Adele was prescribed an antacid called Ranitidine.

As a holistic mother and a health counselor, I knew all this drug would do was to suppress some of the pain while creating new symptoms — aka "side effects." I knew the medication would not eliminate the reason why Adele was getting sick, and it wouldn't cure her.

I decided to take a couple of weeks and try treating Adele with natural remedies, such as herbs, essential oils, and supplements. It seemed logical to me that the stress of starting a new full-time school and being away from me for so long for the first time in her life was triggering her symptoms.

The homeopathic stress-relief remedies I gave Adele helped her to relax, but she was far from being healed. In fact, she was getting worse and was becoming even more afraid to leave the house for fear that the pain would come back.

At this point I was willing to do all that was needed to help her get rid of the symptoms. Between the two "evils," I picked the one I thought was the least: I gave her the drug that her doctors prescribed. I hoped it would reduce her pain and keep her from becoming more socially "disabled."

We gave it a good try, but after two weeks, she wasn't getting better. In fact, she seemed to be getting worse. On top of that, after seeing that the drug had no effect, she was now convinced that nothing could help her. I took her off the drug. For the next two weeks, we went through a rebound effect, that to me felt like what drug addicts must go through while trying to get clean. Taking an antacid makes the body reliant on the drug to stabilize its acid levels. For Adele, this meant that the drug worsened her stomach's natural functioning. Needless to say, it was a painful two-week experience that no child — and no mom — should have to go through.

Our next step was a trip to Boston Children's Hospital, where Adele was seen by a Harvard-trained GI doctor. She was ordered to undergo more tests and was prescribed yet another acid depressant drug, Prilosec (taken by about 70 percent of American adults who are suffering from heartburn). However, this time I knew I wasn't going to put my daughter on yet another precarious drug.

According to the conventional route, our next step would have been to put Adele through an endoscopy procedure to confirm the diagnosis. While this is relatively safe, it does involve placing a tube with the camera into the child's stomach under general anesthesia — always carrying an unpredicted risk for the little patient.

It isn't widely known, but for a child to safely undergo anesthesia, he or she must be clear from colds or any condition causing a stuffed nose for three to four weeks prior to the procedure. During a flu season, this is close to impossible.

It's one thing when a procedure is lifesaving, and quite another when it's an elective case that doesn't guarantee any results, or even the right diagnosis. I just knew this would not be the right or helpful thing to do.

As a holistic health practitioner, I hear a lot of stories from people with food sensitivities. Gluten repeatedly comes up as a common cause of digestive problems. However, since Adele tested negative for gluten sensitivity, I didn't think removing it from her diet would help. But my options were running out and I had nothing to lose, so I decided to take Adele off gluten for a week and see if anything changed.

I did my food shopping over the weekend and on Sunday I took away the bread and pasta. Instead we had gluten-free bread, which Adele loved, and switched to gluten free pasta, which was a great substitution. So I'd say I eliminated about 85 percent of gluten-containing foods from her diet that day.

The very next day, on Monday, I picked Adele up from school and for the first time in months, she didn't burst into tears while telling me how she felt during her heartburn "attacks." Instead she was telling me how good and productive her day was and how she studied and played with her classmates. When I asked if she had any pain, she got quiet for a minute, thinking. And then she said with an astonishing realization, "You know mommy I didn't have any pain today, I forgot all about it."

On Tuesday we had the same wonderful pain-free day. On Wednesday I didn't even ask, and by looking at my daughter's happy, smiling face I knew that she had a great day at school with no destructive pain.

Now, over a year-and-a-half later, Adele is a pain-free, happy child just as a girl her age should be. We continue to be very careful with gluten-containing products. I'd say we're 95 percent gluten free, and that works for us. I can now see that my entire family was affected by this change in our diets.

Switching to gluten-free breads and pastas has allowed me and my husband to feel more energized. My parents, who stocked up on gluten-free foods so that they could feed their visiting grandchildren, also noticed dramatic changes in the condition of their skin. My father's psoriasis skin lesions started to improve, and my mother's skin looks younger and smoother.

The noteworthy fact is that most of my family members are physicians, including my husband and my mother. However, being trained in a conventional medicine system, they would never have imagined that making a small, simple change in one's diet might bring such powerful results.

There are thousands of children (and adults) who experience the same pain that my daughter did. Many of them will undergo unnecessary procedures, only to be left suffering from the symptoms and accepting them as part of their lives.

I know there is another mother right now looking for a way to help her child. I want her to be aware that her solution could be unexpectedly simple and surprisingly inexpensive — just as it was for my daughter.

---

*"It's my passion to inspire and empower people through my seminars, retreats, and private coaching programs. By showing others how to honor their body's wisdom and develop lifelong healthy habits, I help them attain vibrant health, beautiful bodies and boundless energy."*
*— Irene (www.IreneHealthAndWellnessEducator.com)*

## *Non-Celiac Gluten Sensitivity Facts*

You don't test positive for celiac disease
but still react badly to gluten

*"What most people don't know is that gluten can cause serious health complications for many. You may be at risk even if you don't have full blown celiac disease...The problems with wheat are real, scientifically validated and ever-present. Getting off wheat may not only make you feel better and lose weight, it could save your life."*
— *Mark Hyman, MD*

**What Is Non-Celiac Gluten Sensitivity?**
The term non-celiac gluten sensitivity describes those individuals who cannot tolerate gluten and experience symptoms similar to those with celiac disease. They lack the same antibodies and suffer from intestinal damage as seen in celiac disease. Early research suggests that non-celiac gluten sensitivity is an innate immune response, as opposed to an adaptive immune response (such as autoimmune) or allergic reaction.

**Warning Signs and Symptoms**
There are over 250 symptoms of gluten sensitivity that have been reported. Below are the most common ones:
- Bloating
- Abdominal discomfort or pain
- Diarrhea
- Constipation
- Muscular disturbances
- Headaches, migraines
- Severe acne
- Fatigue
- Bone or joint pain
- Headaches

**Statistics**
18 million Americans have gluten sensitivity.
*(That's six times the amount of Americans who have celiac disease.)*

**Further Resources and Helpful Websites**
National Foundation for Celiac Awareness (www.celiaccentral.org)
WebMD.com

# Part II

## Autoimmune Disorders

*2*

## *Celebrating Every Day Together*

*"You can set yourself up to be sick, or you can choose to stay well."*
— *Wayne Dyer*

---

### "Broken" Pancreas

Arlene awakens with a start. Her alarm clock reads 2:00 a.m. She glances at the shadows of her bedroom. Her husband is sleeping soundly next to her. Why is she awake?

The house is quiet except for Nick's rhythmic breathing. Something isn't right. She pulls herself closer and notices his skin is cool and damp. She gently shakes him for quick reassurance that he's okay. Then harder as he doesn't respond. When his eyes finally open, Nick's face is blank. He doesn't recognize her. Arlene doesn't panic. And she doesn't call 911. She simply hurries to the kitchen for juice.

### Live and Learn

When Arlene met Nick, she felt an almost instant connection to him. He felt it too, and they fell madly in love. Three months later, Nick sat Arlene down and said he needed to confess something. He told her of an illness he had that might cut his life short. He didn't know how long he had before his eyesight would deteriorate. How long before he would be bound to a wheelchair. How long he would live. He suffered from type 1 diabetes, and it was not going well.

Nick told her this to give her an out. In spite of his love for her, he would understand if she wanted to leave him. Arlene was devastated. But she came to the decision that even if her time with Nick were to be cut short to a couple of years, she'd take it — they'd make the most of it and celebrate each day they had together.

When Nick was 12, contending with all the confusion and physical changes that come with puberty, he developed an increased thirst. Drinking more fluids was followed, of course, by frequent urination. He also developed a major sweet tooth.

Growing up in New York City, in a neighborhood with poor access to health care, it took Nick many visits to multiple doctors to finally come up with a diagnosis: he had diabetes. At that time, his physicians really didn't understand what was driving the disease. They were not encouraging about his long-term prognosis. He was told not to expect to live a long life. Nick remembers being told, "Don't get used to walking because you're probably going to have a foot amputated."

Nick met Arlene when he was thirty-four. He didn't know it at the time, but he was about to embark upon a lifelong journey of education and healing.

After Nick told Arlene about his illness, she became determined to fully understand diabetes and learn more about ways to treat it. She began researching medical journals and health publications, as well as speaking with Nick's physicians. Over time, she and Nick came to the conclusion that standard treatment was unlikely to provide much help beyond simple insulin injections, which Nick was dependent on: his pancreas was barely functioning. So they shifted their focus to finding ways to better manage Nick's glucose level, which meant carefully choosing the foods he ate.

Throughout this, they concentrated on trying to find the best doctors available to teach them how to better manage the disease. This was easier said than done. They found several experts who appeared to be advanced pioneers in the study of diabetes, but they weren't closely connected to the medical community, and their services — thousands of dollars' worth, it turned out — weren't covered by insurance.

Things started looking up, however, when they made an appointment to see a new physician who came highly recommended. Dr. Bernstein suffered from type 1 diabetes himself, and he made Nick and Arlene feel that they were finally getting the answers they had been searching for.

Dr. Bernstein's approach to living life with diabetes was extremely strict. He expected Nick to follow a regimented diet and test his glucose levels five to eight times each day. The strict diet proscribed by Dr. Bernstein helps his patients achieve constant, near-normal blood glucose levels. This is nothing short of miraculous for many diabetics — but if you want to eat fruit and enjoy occasional sweets, it might not be for you. Thus, the diet made a lot of sense to Nick, but it didn't work with his personality. It didn't fit with his and Arlene's life style, where they tried to make every day as joyful as possible. After two years of working closely with Dr. Bernstein and learning as much as possible from him, Nick stopped seeing him, and he and Arlene have been self-medicating ever since.

It's important to note that they didn't go at it blindly: Nick actually studied medicine at Harvard Medical School before leaving to becoming a computer engineer. His training and interest in medicine helped him determine which tests needed to be performed to monitor his condition. Arlene, on the other hand, is completely self-educated. She developed her expertise through tenacity: constantly asking questions and looking for the answers.

Together, they began to manage Nick's illness systematically — by addressing each part of his body that was not functioning well. In most cases, they were able to treat him by diet alone, including supplements. They discovered, for instance, that asparagus extract was effective in healing Nick's kidneys. Aloe Vera did amazing things for his digestive track.

**A Backward Glance**
Some decisions were easy to make. Others were harder, such as when Nick began to suffer from diabetic retinopathy, a complication of diabetes that affects the eyes. It's caused by damage to the blood vessels of the light-sensitive tissue of the retina, and it's the leading cause of blindness. Diabetic retinopathy often requires a prompt surgical procedure with laser treatment. While surgery can slow or stop the progression of diabetic retinopathy, it's not a cure. Because diabetes is a lifelong condition, eventual vision loss loomed in Nick's future.

Arlene's research into diabetic retinopathy led them to decide against having Nick undergo the operation. She learned about a supplement called astaxanthin. This keto-carotenoid is a powerful antioxidant and free- radical fighter that kills cancer cells. It has to be eaten as a supplement, as we cannot get enough of it through food. After adding astaxanthin to Nick's diet, the progression of damage to his eyes stopped. And what's more, his vision has improved over the last eight years since he started taking it.

Despite Nick and Arlene's success in finding solutions for Nick's diabetes on their own, they continue to work with specialists within the diabetes world. However, they often find that physicians are put off by patients with their level of education and savvy about diabetes. And a few have been downright uncomfortable with them as patients.

At one appointment, a specialist asked Arlene to step out of the office and wait in the waiting room until Nick's examination was over. When pressed by Nick, he revealed that he felt couples tended to not take his sessions seriously when they're together. That was their last visit to him.

The doctor they've stayed with the longest — 14 years and counting works with Arlene and Nick as a member of their team. She runs the tests that they request, and they do what she asks to keep Nick performing well on his annual physical tests.

**Celebrating Each Day**
After 20 years of managing an illness, after the ups and downs of marriage and growing older, after the birth of three beautiful children — Nick and Arlene continue to enjoy the remarkable and inspiring life that Arlene promised herself they'd have. Today Nick is 53 years old, and you could hardly guess that he's older than 35. He feels the same, if not better, than when he met Arlene 20 years ago. His upgraded eyesight is a testament to his improved health.

Together, he and Arlene have become a powerful team, battling his disease and fighting for a happy, fulfilled life together. However, they face constant reminders that Nick's diabetes has not been vanquished. He must be vigilant about checking his blood glucose level and taking insulin to compensate for the food he's eaten. And it's easy to slip up, such as the time he intended to eat an extra piece of dessert and then didn't. He had already compensated for it by injecting extra insulin. After going to bed that evening, the insulin continued to work in his bloodstream, removing the sugar from his body. If Arlene hadn't woken up and noticed that something didn't seem normal — and hadn't known how to get more sugar into his system — the outcome could have been much worse.

This is their reality, and they live their lives one day at a time, while being aware and mindful. Nick knows that if Arlene is not around, such as on a business trip, he has to be more vigilant about not overcompensating with too much insulin.

Currently, there's no cure for type 1 diabetes. Nick's only option to live without depending on insulin injections would be to get a new pancreas. Both he and Arlene stay on top of the latest research and progress in the science behind developing new pancreases.

Arlene credits the medical system for leading her down the path she's taken in life, forcing her to question everything and not give up until she's satisfied with an answer. After a life filled with determination and commitment, courage and devotion, joy and happiness, Arlene and Nick can hardly believe they've been together for as long as they have. Their marriage, like Nick's health, is going strong. After 20 years, they're still in love and still celebrating every day they spend together.

---

*"It's your life and your health, own it and thrive. Using food as a preventative form of medicine, along with healthy lifestyle choices, we can achieve and maintain health and wellness."*

*— Arlene (www.arlenefigueroa.com)*

# *Type 1 Diabetes Facts*

*"There's no known way to prevent type 1 diabetes. But researchers are working on preventing the disease or further destruction of the islet cells in people who are newly diagnosed."*
*— Mayo Clinic*

**What Is Type 1 Diabetes (T1D)?**
If a person is diagnosed with type 1 diabetes, their pancreas produces little to no insulin; their body's immune system destroys the insulin-producing cells in the pancreas.

**How Is T1D Managed?**
People with the disease must carefully balance insulin doses (either by injections multiple times a day or continuous infusion through a pump) with eating and other activities throughout the day and night. They must measure their blood-glucose level by pricking their fingers for blood six or more times a day, as they always run the risk of dangerous high or low blood-glucose levels, both of which can be life threatening.

**Warning Signs and Symptoms**
- Extreme thirst
- Frequent urination
- Drowsiness and lethargy
- Sugar in urine
- Sudden vision changes
- Increased appetite
- Sudden weight loss
- Fruity, sweet, or wine-like odor on breath
- Heavy, labored breathing
- Stupor or unconsciousness

**Statistics**
- As many as three million Americans may have T1D.
- Each year, more than 15,000 children and 15,000 adults — approximately 80 people per day — are diagnosed with T1D in the U.S.
- Approximately 85 percent of people living with T1D are adults, and 15 percent of people living with T1D are children.

- The rate of T1D incidence among children under age 14 is estimated to increase by three percent annually worldwide.
- T1D accounts for $14.9 billion in healthcare costs in the U.S. each year.

**Further Resources and Helpful Websites**

Juvenile Diabetes Research Foundation (jdrf.org)

*3*
## *Living with Rheumatoid Arthritis:*
## *How to Thrive and Be Healthy*

*"Pain insists upon being attended to. God whispers to us in our pleasures, speaks in our consciences, but shouts in our pains. It is his megaphone to rouse a deaf world."*
— *C.S. Lewis*

In her early twenties, Barbara took up high-impact aerobics. Like many women her age, she wanted to look and feel better. But before long she had to stop. The exercises caused her back to curve in an uncomfortable way, and instead of feeling better, she felt worse.

Soon she felt pain when she simply sat at her desk at work. She found relief with low-impact exercise and regular visits to a chiropractor. A few years later, while downhill skiing, Barbara fell on the slopes and injured her right knee. After she recovered, she was still in chronic pain — and she could no longer continue with her exercises. She started to feel depressed and quickly began to understand the connection between chronic pain and mental health.

Barbara's doctors couldn't determine what was wrong because her pain wasn't consistent. Finally they agreed to perform orthoscopic surgery to investigate the condition of her knee more closely. Behind her kneecap, they discovered a piece of cartilage about the size of a dime, which hadn't shown up on any of the previous imaging. They removed it, and Barbara was able to get back to her exercise routine, which helped stabilize her knee and lift her depression.

With her new-found mobility, Barbara decided to make major changes in her life. She became more diligent about getting regular exercise. She improved her diet. She gave up her stressful, career in the high-pressure world of advertising. She went back to school and became a successful, full-time massage therapist.

### Getting a Diagnosis
Six years later, Barbara started experiencing pain again. This time it was in her hands, the very tools she used to give massages. She was

devastated. In addition, her favorite shoes began to feel uncomfortable at the end of her workday. The joints in her feet ached, and she got so tired during the day that she couldn't continue her exercise routine.

Barbara tried to alleviate the pain and swelling on her own by using massage techniques. But they didn't get better. And a few months later — just three days before her 45th birthday — she was finally diagnosed with rheumatoid arthritis.

At the time, Barbara was giving about twenty-five massages a week. Determined to not lose her livelihood to her disease, she found a new rheumatologist. He not only treated her physical condition, but also supported her emotionally. He encouraged her to not give up the profession she loved, as that would mean giving up something that made her who she was. He reassured her that she could fight and, eventually, beat the disease while continuing to do what was making her happy.

With the support and guidance of her new rheumatologist, she got better. After only eighteen months, Barbara was in remission. And she did it without cutting back on her massage therapy clients, taking the smallest doses of medicine possible, and refusing to give up her high heels.

**Barbara's Techniques for Thriving with Rheumatoid Arthritis**
So what was it that Barbara did to beat rheumatoid arthritis and eventually heal? Here are her healing strategies:
- She *did* take medications, but the lowest doses possible (no NSAIDs, prednisone, or biologics)
- She ate primarily whole, non-processed, home-cooked foods
- She went from minimizing wheat to being completely gluten free
- She did yoga and water exercises at least two or three times a week
- She made sure to get plenty of sleep and relaxation

Below are some additional techniques Barbara developed to speed her recovery and minimize pain.

Actions she took with her body:
- Got up and moved at least once each hour during the day
- Sat cross-legged for five or ten minutes daily to gently stretch her hips
- Avoided putting her shoulders on the pillow when sleeping (as this over-stretched the muscles in her upper back); rather, she

slept with her shoulders flat, giving her muscles a better chance to relax

- Sat outside with her shoes off and put her feet in the grass for ten minutes each day — she felt this "earthing" routine decreased her pain and inflammation through balancing her body's electrical charge with the earth's
- Found a massage therapist who specialized in chronic pain and had a massage at least once every eight weeks

What she ate:

- High-quality fish oil on a daily basis to help balance any inflammatory fats in her body
- Liquids to stay hydrated, which made a tremendous difference in helping her muscles and joints function properly
- Leafy green vegetables for their natural detoxification effect on the body

What she did not eat:

- Trans fats, as they are a major contributor to pain and inflammation
- Sugar (as little as possible), as it increases the body's fluid retention - often a factor in pain and stiffness

Barbara finds that living with rheumatoid arthritis takes creating a sort of tightrope balance in her life. There are days when she feels like swinging freely, and there are days when she just tries to stay on her feet and not fall. Since Barbara knows first-hand how to live and thrive with rheumatoid arthritis, she now helps other entrepreneurs get in control of their pain so they don't need to give up living full lives and managing their businesses.

---

*"Health-coaching people — who, like me, are both entrepreneurs and have chronic pain is now my mission."*

— *Barbara (www.confidentwellness.com)*

# *Rheumatoid Arthritis (RA) Facts*

*"Pain, especially chronic pain, is an emotional condition as well as a physical sensation. It is a complex experience that affects thought, mood, and behavior and can lead to isolation, immobility, and drug dependence."*
*— Harvard Health Publications, Harvard Medical School*

**What Is Rheumatoid Arthritis?**
Rheumatoid arthritis is an autoimmune disease in which your body's immune system — which protects your health by attacking foreign substances like bacteria and viruses — mistakenly attacks your joints. The abnormal immune response causes inflammation that can damage joints and organs, such as the heart.

**Warning Signs and Symptoms**
- Tender, warm, swollen joints
- Morning stiffness that may last for hours
- Firm bumps of tissue under the skin on your arms (rheumatoid nodules)
- Fatigue
- Fever
- Weight loss

Early rheumatoid arthritis tends to affect the smaller joints first, particularly the joints that attach your fingers to your hands and your toes to your feet. When the disease progresses, symptoms may spread to the knees, ankles, elbows, hips, and shoulders.

**Statistics**
- About 0.6% of the United States adult population has RA (about
- 1.5 million people)
- Women are two to three times as likely to have RA as men
- Onset is most frequent during middle age, but people of any age can be affected

**Further Resources and Helpful Websites**
Arthritis Foundation (www.arthritistoday.org)

# 4
# *Kaitlyn's Search for Diagnosis,*
# *Cure and the Recovery of Her Life*

*"The body is one integrated system, not a collection of organs divided up by medical specialties. The medicine of the future connects everything."*
— *Mark Hyman, M.D.*

"From Pain Comes Strength" was the title of Kaitlyn's college application essay. If you met her on campus of Northeastern University, where she attends a Physical Therapy graduate program, you'd never guess that within that happy, healthy young woman lies an arduous back-story filled with debilitating pain and courageous strength.

Kaitlyn led a fairly normal childhood. She suffered from chronic ear infections and psoriasis, but never anything more severe than that. One night, when she was 11, she awoke in the middle of the night in extreme pain. She came to her parents' room for help, unable to stand upright. Right away her parents took her to the emergency room. The attending physician performed standard tests, but couldn't determine what was causing the pain, other than a suspicion that her appendix was involved. In the morning, Kaitlyn was released from the hospital with a prescription for pain medication — but no diagnosis.

The next day Kaitlyn's mother, Debbie, took her to see their pediatrician. He also couldn't find what was wrong and couldn't account for the extreme pain. Kaitlyn's blood tests didn't reveal anything, and the pediatrician suggested they wait and see how her condition progressed. From that moment forward, Kaitlyn experienced constant pain — until two-and-a- half years later, when she found an alternative route to recovery.

## Hard Questions
Initially, Kaitlyn described her discomfort as somebody kicking her in the stomach. It was severe pain, localized in the left, lower part of her stomach. Later, she felt the same pain throughout her body, particularly in her wrists, hands, and knees. She began to develop arthritis.

Kaitlyn went through extensive testing: CAT scans, x-rays, and

21

everything in between. Throughout this, her condition worsened. She began experiencing bowel issues, including diarrhea and constipation. She had difficulty sleeping.

Six weeks after making her way to her parents' bedroom, from that initial outburst of pain, Kaitlyn found she was not able to get out of bed. Her pain was excruciating. Her hands were so "prickly" that she couldn't move them. She couldn't even hold a pen.

Her primary-care doctor was at a loss and suggested that they might be dealing with a psychological issue. He arranged for Kaitlyn to see a psychologist. Debbie took her to the appointment and was surprised when she was asked to wait in a different room. She agreed, thinking they were simply going to do more blood work.

In the car, after the appointment, Kaitlyn began crying. She said that the psychologist accused her of pretending to be sick and laughed at her. He asked if she was a lesbian. She was as confused and scared, as any 13-year- old would be. Debbie was also confused. And she was discouraged and angry. She knew that she would have to find yet another doctor.

Eventually Kaitlyn was referred to a rheumatologist who prescribed a medication that is usually used for breast cancer. He explained that with low dosages it could help with Kaitlyn's arthritis. With few other options Debbie agreed to try. Soon, Kaitlyn got the use of her hands back, and it gave her the first glimmer of hope.

Throughout this, Kaitlin needed 24-hour care because she couldn't sleep at night, which led to further symptoms and physical problems. Her condition also took an emotional toll, as she wasn't able to go to school and see her friends. Her mom stopped working to care for Kaitlyn throughout the day and tutor her. Kaitlyn's school allowed her to finish seventh grade from home.

### "Why Can't You Figure Anything Out?"
Kaitlyn now had her summer vacation to figure things out, but she still was not getting better. She felt like her doctors were merely experimenting on her, constantly switching her drugs. In one instance, she was put on Enbrel, which is self-injected and usually used to treat long-term inflammatory diseases. Initially, it helped a little with her knees. However, the injections, which had to be put into Kaitlyn's thigh, were painful and traumatizing. One night she experienced a serious reaction.

Just after her injection, she felt like she couldn't breathe and her tongue and face got swollen. At the emergency room, she was told to stop taking it.

Another emergency room visit was prompted by Kaitlyn feeling numbness in her right arm. She also felt severe pain in her chest, and her blood pressure was sky high. However, she was unable to get a clinical diagnosis of what was wrong. Kaitlyn's mother broke down. She exclaimed to the emergency room doctor, "Are these medications killing my daughter? What's going on with her? Why can't you figure anything out?" The response was no different from the previous six times Kaitlyn had been to the ER.

It began to dawn on Debbie that each doctor looked for a cure within their specialty. If they found none, they sent Kaitlyn off to another specialist. It was up to the family to tell each specialist what the other doctors were doing, why they were sent to them, and so on. She saw they weren't working as team — with each other or with Kaitlyn. And no one was looking at the whole picture. This was the moment Debbie knew they needed to find a new direction.

**Holistic Getaway**
The following summer Debbie thought that it would be good for Kaitlyn to get away for a change in surroundings. She sent her to stay with her grandmother, thinking that even if Kaitlyn spent all her time in bed, at least it would be a different bed.

One of the first things Kaitlyn's grandmother did was take her to get her nails and toes done. Kaitlyn was 13 and had never had this done before. In the salon, Kaitlyn spoke to her grandmother about her struggles. They were overheard by a woman who practiced massage in the office along with other holistic practitioners. She suggested that Kaitlyn try massage therapy.

Kaitlyn agreed to give cranio-sacral massage a try, and for the first time in one-and-a-half years she felt amazing. The feeling of being free of pain lasted only 20 minutes, but it gave her hope. Up until then, Kaitlyn's mother followed the direction of traditional doctors. That's all she knew, and it's what she trusted. Even though people had suggested that she check out holistic medicine and massage, Debbie didn't understand how they could help her daughter.

Kaitlyn's next scheduled medical procedure was a colonoscopy. Once again, her doctors didn't learn anything significant. However, a follow-up endoscopy showed that Kaitlyn was lactose intolerant and didn't have any of the lactase enzymes. She was ordered to take an antinuclear antibody test, which is a primary test to help evaluate a person for autoimmune disorders. She tested positive. Finally, discovering that Kaitlyn had a type of autoimmune disease felt like they had unlocked the first piece of the puzzle. However, no one could say how it related to the whole picture of all her symptoms.

Now Debbie was ready to call the massage therapist back. Kaitlin had her second treatment and, once again, had the same reaction of being completely pain free. This owner of the practice had a background in medicine and was now practicing holistic and functional medicine. He felt there was more to healing that traditional medicine could offer, and got his start helping his own family. Soon he became a Chinese herbalist. He agreed to treat Kaitlyn.

He explained to Debbie that applying traditional acupuncture might cause pain for Kaitlin, as she was too sensitive, and it would have been too much for her body. He instead did an uncommon kind of acupuncture called shakuju therapy. During the procedure, Kaitlyn vomited in the office, but she felt amazing afterward.

The doctor also checked Kaitlyn's blood and determined that she had candida. He suggested that she remove sugar and gluten from her diet. He put her on probiotics. This was the first her family had heard about their healing power. The doctor suspected that the antibiotics used to treat Kaitlyn's previous ear infections might have contributed to what she was going through now. She did not have enough good bacteria in her gut, as most of it was likely killed by antibiotics and was never restored.

Within two months of going through these new treatments, Kaitlin felt terrific. She was sleeping at night, which was one of the most important accomplishments, as she couldn't heal if she was not sleeping. And she was able to go back to school.

Kaitlyn still had constant pain in her chest that her doctors couldn't explain. Back at the practice, she saw the physical therapist, who discovered that Kaitlin had an extra set of ribs, known as floating ribs. He said he could "pop" the ribs in right there. While Debbie was a little weary of that, as it still was new to her, she saw that they had nothing to lose. After all, these people gave her daughter the support she never had before. Kaitlyn and Debbie trusted them. And sure enough, the physical therapist popped back in Kaitlyn's ribs, exactly where the pain had been. Kaitlin felt amazing.

This was the first time a doctor and all other medical practitioners in the office seemed to genuinely care. They made Debbie and Kaitlyn feel like they were going to work hard to get to the root of the problem. They assured them that they'd helped other patients go through amazing transformations and gave Kaitlyn and her family the confidence that she would heal too. They inspired them to see a beautiful future ahead for Kaitlin, even though nobody else could see it at the time.

The combination of constant encouragement and care with the fact that Kaitlyn was feeling less pain was life changing just as it was lifesaving. When Kaitlyn was sixteen, a woman who had a sick child asked her about her story. To everybody's amazement, Kaitlin said that getting sick was the best thing that could ever happen to her because now she knows her purpose in life. She wants to help other people and do all she can to ensure that no one has to go through the pain that she did.

**The Trick Is Awareness**
Today Kaitlyn is almost 20. She is in her second year of a physical therapy program. Looking back, it's hard for her to believe that she went from being in constant debilitating pain for over two years to being able play lacrosse.

She feels great and takes care of herself so she can stay healthy. She exercises, practices yoga, and meditates. Her rib still pops out occasionally. But now she knows exactly what it is and how to deal with it.

For Kaitlyn, the key part of keeping healthy is her diet. Keeping gluten out of her diet has made a huge difference in her health. Cutting down on sugar seems to have had the biggest effect. Being a normal teenager and college student, she slips up sometimes, such as eating pasta with friends. She keeps on a strict diet for three to four days a week, and then may allow herself to indulge a little. However, the trick is that now she can recognize when she's starting to feel bad and fix herself right away.

Kaitlyn goes to regular checkups at the Integrative Health Medical Center. She takes probiotics religiously, which help maintain beneficial bacteria in her bowels. There are few more essential supplements she takes including omegas, multivitamins, B12, and D3.

She takes no medications and feels thankful to not have pain and to be able to enjoy life. After more than two years of searching for a diagnosis and a cure, once she found the alternative route, it took about six months before she really got to a place where she was feeling great.

Kaitlyn's family also changed. After seeing her suffer after taking countless medications and then not get any better, their position on holistic medicine changed dramatically.

**A Look Back**
When Kaitlyn felt fully recovered, she went back to see the rheumatologist they had consulted with at the onset of her symptoms, who wasn't able to determine what was going on with her. Kaitlyn and Debbie stayed up the night before their visit, writing down the steps they took that helped get her to a diagnosis and find a cure. Trying to make sure they didn't miss any important detail from Kaitlyn's recuperation, they brought all the records and the x-rays, so that this doctor could use them to effectively help his other patients with similar symptoms.

The doctor was shocked, and his first reaction was that there was no way Kaitlyn was the same girl he saw almost two years ago. She felt and looked amazing and had no signs of arthritis in her knees or hands. Then he stunned them both by declining to learn more. He simply said, *"I don't need to see any of this. It sounds like you're doing fine so you don't need me."*

Kaitlyn and Debbie were disappointed but not discouraged. After over two years of desperately searching for the answers, they value their education that made them empowered patients. They know enough to choose doctors who care and can see patients as more than their illness. They know that great doctors are true healers and heroes who do their best to find out the root cause of your problems and guide you through each step to your recovery.

---

*"I'm just a mother who went through a great ordeal and hope that our story will help other moms and their kids avoid that. As a parent who lived through their child's illness I wish we had the book like that back then."*

*— Debbie*

# Psoriatic Arthritis and Cervical Rib/Thoracic Outlet Syndrome Facts

*"Over 90 percent of the population suffers from inflammation or an autoimmune disorder. Until now, conventional medicine has said there is no cure. Minor irritations like rashes and runny noses are ignored, while chronic and debilitating diseases like Crohn's and rheumatoid arthritis are handled with a cocktail of toxic treatments that fail to address their root cause. But it doesn't have to be this way."*
— *Dr. Amy Myers, MD*

## What Is Psoriatic Arthritis?

Psoriatic arthritis is a form of arthritis that affects some people who have psoriasis, which is a condition that features red patches of skin topped with silvery scales. The vast majority of people develop psoriasis first and are later diagnosed with psoriatic arthritis, however, the joint problems can begin before skin lesions appear.

## Warning Signs and Symptoms

Psoriatic arthritis can affect joints on just one side or on both sides of your body. The signs and symptoms of psoriatic arthritis often resemble those of rheumatoid arthritis as both diseases cause joints to become painful, swollen, and warm to the touch. Psoriatic arthritis is more likely to cause:

- Swollen fingers and toes
- Foot pain
- Lower back pain

## Statistics

Up to 30 percent of people with psoriasis develop psoriatic arthritis. Psoriatic arthritis affects as many as 750,000 people in the United States alone. It can develop at any time, but it most commonly appears between the ages of 30 and 50.

## What is Cervical Rib/Thoracic Outlet Syndrome?

At the back, this rib connects to the seventh cervical vertebra in the neck. At the front, in some people a cervical rib can be 'floating' and have no connection. In other people it can be connected to their first rib by a band of tough, fibrous tissue. In some others there may be an articulation (like in a joint) with their first rib.

27

The thoracic outlet is a space, or passageway, that lies just above the first rib and behind the collarbone (clavicle) and it runs from the base of the neck to the armpit.

## Statistics

- About 1 in 200 people are born with an extra rib called a cervical rib.
- About 1 in 10 people who have a cervical rib develop thoracic outlet syndrome.
- The thoracic outlet syndrome is more common in women than in men and it can occur from the ages of 20 to 80, but is most common around the age of 40.

## Further Resources and Helpful Websites

National Psoriasis Foundation (www.psoriasis.org)
Mayo Clinic (www.mayoclinic.org)
Patient.co.uk

# 5

## *How Ellen Overcame Celiac Disease and Alopecia: Becoming The Radiant and Vibrant Woman She Was Meant to Be*

*"The most serious form of allergy to gluten, celiac disease, affects one in 100 people, or three million Americans, most of who don't know they have it."*
— *Mark Hyman, MD*

From as early as Ellen could remember, she had frequent stomachaches, primarily after she ate. It didn't matter what or where she ate, she often suffered terrible bloating afterward. And she blamed herself, believing that it was caused by her lack of self-control and overeating. She beat herself up over this, disappointed that she couldn't control herself when it came to food. The anguish she felt wreaked havoc on her emotions. And while she didn't know it at the time, damage was also being done to the inside of her body.

In March of 2005, Ellen's hairdresser told her that she noticed bald patches on her scalp. Ellen sought help from a specialist, searching for an explanation. She found the first dermatologist she spoke with to be somewhat patronizing. She was told to simply calm down, that eventually her hair would grow back. She made an appointment to see another dermatologist, and it went the same way.

Not ready to give up, she saw a third doctor, who performed a hormonal test and diagnosed Ellen with alopecia, an autoimmune disease that affects the hair follicles. Beyond that, there were few explanations about the cause, other than it might have been caused by a virus. The dermatologist recommended that he inject cortisone into her bare scalp as a possible cure — but he offered no guarantee. And even if it worked, her hair might fall out again. She might lose it in other places too.

Even though her third doctor was her hero for being willing to do the necessary testing, Ellen decided to hold off on his recommendation and investigate her condition on her own.

**Against the Grain**
Ellen read everything on alopecia that she could get her hands on. After

29

nine months of research, she came across a book called "Dangerous Grains." In it, the author, Dr. Ron Hoggan, made a strong argument for a connection between celiac disease and a wide array of autoimmune diseases, including alopecia. Ellen immediately called her internist and asked for a celiac blood test.

One of Ellen's sisters had been diagnosed with celiac disease about six years earlier, but her doctor never suggested that the rest of her family be tested. Ellen's blood test came back positive. She was notified of the news by a dry, formal letter. There was no phone call, no appointment, and no information about what gluten was or how to give it up. Thankfully, her sister had already figured out a way to live gluten free without it destroying her will to live. For Ellen, it turned her life upside down.

In November 2005, Ellen began eating a gluten-free diet. In the middle of that month, on a business trip, she called her sister at least a million times for help and advice, trying her best to maintain a gluten-free diet. She returned home frustrated and depressed. How would she travel? How would she entertain guests at home? How would she go to other people's homes for dinner?

Ellen's internist initially told her that she didn't need to have an endoscopy to confirm the diagnosis of celiac disease. But she scheduled one anyway* with the head of the Celiac Clinic at Beth Israel Hospital in Boston. She wanted to know the extent of her intestinal damage. She wanted to know, beyond the blood-test results, why she needed to follow a gluten-free diet.

The test confirmed that she had scalloped intestines, a certain sign of celiac disease. Her doctors also confirmed that she would need to be on a strict gluten-free diet for the rest of her life. This time Ellen knew she had to commit herself to it.

**Better Food, Better Mood**
Three years after going completely gluten free, the hair on the back of Ellen's scalp completely returned. The hair loss next to her ear grew back 75 percent. Her stomach discomfort became rare, except when she overate or inadvertently eat gluten. Ellen saw further improvements when she significantly cut back on dairy, about a year into being gluten free.

Now she eats an almost completely plant-based, non-animal diet. While she never in a million years thought she'd give up eating flesh, she found it works for her. Ellen feels like a new person, she likes who she has become. And the rest of her family does too. Her mood fluctuations have all but disappeared, replaced by a steady, calm demeanor — and a fierce desire to cook and bake.

Ellen used to love bagels and crusty French bread. She now bakes them herself without using gluten. She has found gluten-free restaurants that she likes, admitting that gluten free at one place isn't necessarily the same as the next. Some will go to great lengths, while others simply say that they have gluten-free menu items, but they don't seem to fully understand what it takes to offer safe gluten-free food to customers.

In case of slip-ups, Ellen has found remedies that help, including Doterra Essential Oil blend Digestzen, and charcoal — both effective if she inadvertently eats gluten. Also, she applies Super Lysine on canker sores, a common side effect of celiac disease.

While being gluten free of course poses some challenges, for Ellen the benefits far outweigh the disadvantages. In the past, she was bloated, irritable, moody, and exhausted. Now, the bloat has disappeared, her moods have evened out, and she's rarely exhausted. Most of what Ellen knows, she learned from trial and error, books, and others with celiac disease. She's also grateful for online support forums, which connect her with others and help her to not feel so alone.

After ten years, Ellen's hair is mostly back, with just a few thin spots. And she even has a solution for that in the form of an excellent hairdresser.

---

*"I am passionate about helping people transition to a way of gluten-free eating that will help them fall in love with the food that loves them back."*
— *Ellen (www.glutenfreediva.com)*

*\*Please note: This advice is not recommended for the general public. If you've been diagnosed with celiac disease, you don't necessarily need an endoscopy. This was Ellen's personal choice.*

# *Celiac Disease Facts*

*"There's good, solid evidence of an overlap between celiac disease and other autoimmune disorders."*
*— Harvard Medical School Health Publications*

## What Is Celiac Disease?

Celiac disease is a digestive and autoimmune disorder that results in damage to the lining of the small intestine when foods with gluten are eaten *(Glutens are a form of protein found in some grains)*. As a result, the damage to the intestine makes it hard for the body to absorb nutrients, especially fat, calcium, iron, and folate.

## Warning Signs and Symptoms

(may vary)

- Digestive problems (abdominal bloating, pain, gas, diarrhea, pale stools, and weight loss)
- Severe skin rash called dermatitis herpetiformis
- Iron deficiency anemia (low blood count)
- Musculoskeletal problems (muscle cramps, joint and bone pain)
- Growth problems and failure to thrive (in children)
- Seizures
- Tingling sensation in the legs (caused by nerve damage and low calcium)
- Aphthous ulcers (sores in the mouth)
- Missed menstrual periods

Celiac disease can leave a person susceptible to other health problems, including:

- Osteoporosis, a disease that weakens bones and leads to fractures
- Miscarriage or infertility
- Birth defects, such as neural tube defects (improper formation of the spine)
- Seizures
- Growth problems in children
- Cancer of the intestine (very rare)

People who have celiac disease may have other autoimmune diseases, including:

- Thyroid disease
- Type 1 diabetes
- Lupus
- Rheumatoid arthritis
- Sjögren's syndrome (a disorder that causes insufficient moisture production by the glands)

Undiagnosed or untreated celiac disease can lead to:
- Iron deficiency anemia
- Early onset osteoporosis or osteopenia
- Infertility and miscarriage
- Lactose intolerance
- Vitamin and mineral deficiencies
- Central and peripheral nervous system disorders
- Pancreatic insufficiency
- Intestinal lymphomas and other GI cancers (malignancies)
- Gall bladder malfunction
- Neurological manifestations, including ataxia, epileptic seizures, dementia, migraine, neuropathy, myopathy and multifocal leucoencephalopathy

**Statistics**
- Celiac disease is thought to affect 1 in 100 people worldwide.
- 2.5 million Americans are undiagnosed and are at risk for long-term health complications

# *Alopecia Areata Facts*

**What Is Alopecia Areata?**
Alopecia areata is a type of hair loss that occurs when your immune system mistakenly attacks hair follicles. The damage to the follicle is usually not permanent.

**Warning Signs and Symptoms**
Alopecia areata often is asymptomatic, however, some patients (14%) experience a burning sensation in the affected area. The condition usually is localized when it first appears, as follows:
- Single patch - 80%
- Two patches - 2.5%
- Multiple patches - 7.7%

No correlation exists between the number of patches at onset and subsequent severity. Alopecia areata can affect any hair-bearing area, and more than one area can be affected at once. Associated conditions may include the following:
- Atopic dermatitis
- Vitiligo
- Thyroid disease
- Collagen-vascular diseases
- Down syndrome
- Psychiatric disorders - Anxiety, personality disorders, depression, and paranoid disorders
- Stressful life events in the six months before onset

**Statistics**
- Alopecia areata affects approximately 2% of the population overall. In the United States more than 6.5 million people are affected.
- Alopecia areata is most common in people younger than 20 and women and men are affected equally.

**Further Resources and Helpful Websites**
Celiac Disease Foundation (celiac.org)
Web MD (www.webmd.com)
National Alopecia Areata Foundation (www.naaf.org)
Medscape (emedicine.medscape.com)

*6*

## *How Jarod Lives and Thrives with Multiple Sclerosis*

*"Men over 50 with multiple sclerosis do not get better. But I am. I am 57, with MS for 29 years. I'm a thriver, not merely a survivor of MS. I'm a victor over it, not a victim of MS. I have it; it will never have me!"*
*— Jarod Jacobs*

Jarod was used to working long hours and had settled into a busy and stressful life. He lived in New York and ran a successful business selling vegetables to restaurants and schools. His schedule left him little time to focus on his health. But one day, he felt off in way that alarmed him: a dullness and tingling in his left shoulder. He didn't know what it was, but he knew something was wrong.

Jarod went to a neurologist who recommended an MRI. The test confirmed his doctor's diagnosis of multiple sclerosis. Jarod had just turned 29. He was told that there was no treatment and no cure for MS. His doctor simply said, "Just go and live your life." So that's what he did. He kept busy running his business. He got married. He moved from New York to Florida.

After many years of living his life, he found his symptoms were worsening. His condition was finally affecting his ability to do his job, and he had to stop working full time. This prompted Jarod to start working more closely with his neurologist.

He tried all the drugs that were out there. Nothing worked, and his symptoms kept worsening. After a few years, his neurologist suggested not to use drugs anymore. At this point, Jarod felt his medications were poison and was glad to stop taking them.

Instead, he made major changes to his diet. He cut down on salt and meat. He took 50 well-researched supplements a day. But over time, it didn't seem to help.

Next, Jarod found an alternative-care facility in Nepal. Over the course of his 28 days there, he became a full-fledged vegetarian. He went to

35

physical therapy. And he learned about the power of attitude. These changes were perfectly aligned with the skills that made his business a success: diligence, never taking a break, always taking care of himself, never cheating or making excuses. His mantra became "You've got to believe that you can, you've got to want to be healthy, you've got to take full responsibility for yourself."

He came away with a new way to live and finally began to feel better. Below are the five changes that made all the difference in Jarod's health.

**1. Raw Vegan Diet**
Jarod approaches food as something fun and enjoyable. At the same time he eats to nourish and replenish his body with the nutrients it needs to function well. He believes that our bodies will achieve their perfect weight if we just provide the right materials. If you follow the right diet, you'll weigh exactly what you're supposed to and can never be too fat or too skinny. Because of his diet, Jarod easily maintains his weight, which is very important for someone with MS.

Here is Jarod's raw vegan diet:
- Lunch: juice, salad, and melon
- Mid-afternoon snack: three oranges
- Dinner: the same as lunch, but with an additional two ounces of seaweed salad
- Evening snack: sweet potato or veggie chips

Jarod's juice:
- 3 bunches of kale (spinach or Swiss chard)
- 2 celery, 2 carrots, 2 cucumbers
- 1 gala apple, 2 bananas
- Spring parsley, spring cilantro
- 2 oz. coconut milk
- 1 tablespoon chia seeds
- Spring mix lettuce
- Red onion
- Red cabbage
- Bella mushroom
- Tomato
- Celery, carrot, cucumber
- Mixed peppers
- Avocado, hemp seed oil
- Himalayan salt and lemon dressing

Jarod's dessert:
- Watermelon, cantaloupe, or pineapple

## 2. Chiropractic Adjustments
Multiple sclerosis is a neurological condition. Since the part of the body that controls the nerves is the spine, a chiropractor's help makes sense to Jarod, and he has been getting the treatments to help his spine work better weekly.

## 3. Physical Therapy
People with MS tire easily and can get flustered when they can't perform certain functions. Physical therapists help develop a specific exercise program based on a patient's condition and goals. Seeing a physical therapist can help with:

Balance problems
Clumsiness and poor coordination
Fatigue
Fitness
Pain
Weakness
Strategies to save energy

## 4. Avoiding Conventional Doctors and Pharmaceuticals
Jarod believes that we have to take responsibility for our own life, and there are times when we can't simply let a doctor tell us what to do. We need to become our own superheroes. Jarod isn't convinced that all doctors really want us to get better, because they don't want to lose us as a patient. Integrative medicine, on the other hand, is the way to go and integrate the mind and the body while looking at the very root of the health issue.

## 5. Maintaining a Great Attitude
Jarod loves that he can be an inspiration for others. He says that he's nowhere near perfect, but he feels so good that he feels guilty. He's 58 years old, and he knows that men at 50 with MS often don't get the chance to be alive to say that. He knows that he is a living miracle and knows that what he is doing is really powerful.

And he looks great. He has no grey hair. His belly is flat. His eyes are sharp. His brain works fine. He attributes all of this to his diet. Jarod hasn't had an MS attack episodes in more than eight years. You can see Jarod's walking progress on YouTube. Search "Jarod walking."

**Important Dates**
- Jarod's MS Diagnosis: 1986
- Jarod stops taking MS drugs: 2007
- Jarod starts eating an organic vegetarian diet: 2009 Jarod goes raw vegan: 2013

---

*"Negative people say, 'It works for you, not everyone.' Positive people say, 'If it works for you, it could work for me.' YAGOTTAWANNA!"*

*— Jarod*

# *Multiple Sclerosis Facts*

*"I had about four days of like, 'Pity party, woe is me, it's all over.' Then I did some research and spoke with doctors and got in contact with people who have MS, and I soon realized it's actually a lot more manageable than the kind of public perception of it is, and that's part of the reason why I've been so outspoken about it."*
*— Jack Osbourne*

### What Is Multiple sclerosis?
Multiple sclerosis (MS) is a disease in which your immune system attacks the protective sheath (myelin) that covers your nerves. Myelin damage disrupts communication between your brain and the rest of your body and ultimately, the nerves themselves may deteriorate, a process that's currently irreversible.

### Warning Signs and Symptoms
Signs and symptoms of multiple sclerosis vary, depending on the location of affected nerve fibers. They may include:
- Numbness or weakness in one or more limbs that typically occurs on one side of your body at a time, or the legs and trunk
- Partial or complete loss of vision, usually in one eye at a time, often with pain during eye movement
- Double vision or blurring of vision
- Tingling or pain in parts of your body
- Electric-shock sensations that occur with certain neck movements, especially bending the neck forward
- Tremor, lack of coordination or unsteady gait
- Slurred speech
- Fatigue
- Dizziness
- Problems with bowel and bladder function

### Statistics
- It's estimated that more than 400,000 people in the United States and about 2.5 million people around the world have MS
- In the United States, about 200 new cases are diagnosed each week.
- Rates of MS are higher farther from the equator

- It's estimated that in southern states (below the 37$^{th}$ parallel), the rate of MS is 57 to 78 cases per 100,000 people
- In northern states (above the 37$^{th}$ parallel), the rate is twice as high, at about 110 to 140 cases per 100,000
- The incidence of MS is also higher in colder climates

**Further Resources and Helpful Websites**

The National MS Society (www.nationalmssociety.org)

# 7
# *Connecting the Dots for*
# *Health and Recovery*

*Getting a handle on autoimmune disorders*

*"Regrettably, we've become a culture that is very dependent on having a quick fix. People are handing their bodies over to outside sources without understanding what, when, where, and why what they are feeling is happening. They just want the symptoms go away. It is time to reclaim our physiology, to salvage our understanding of how our bodies have been impacted by our personal histories and our skills for self-care."*
— *Andrea Nakayama*

Have you ever wished there was a qualified specialist who could guide you through the process of connecting the dots for your health and recovery?

**Meet Andrea Nakayama and her team of functional nutritionists.**
Conventional medical professionals tend to focus on pinpointing a patient's symptoms and then applying a single "cure." Functional nutritionists instead look at your health as a system. They attempt to intimately understand your history, triggering events, lab results, and factors that may contribute to your condition.

As a result, they create a highly effective, custom-tailored treatment plan to meet your health goals. Most work alongside your physician, complementing their skills and abilities. Functional nutritionists not only help you get well, but they also teach you how to be in charge of your own health.

Andrea's typical patient has been to many doctors and has tried just about every treatment that conventional medicine has to offer them. Yet, the physicians they see and the medications they take don't seem to help with their ailments. Finding the correct remedy for these patients takes uncovering the cause of their illness. The level of digging and persistence this requires isn't taught and is rarely practiced within the conventional medical system.

**Andrea's Personal Loss and Healing**
When Andrea was pregnant with her first and only baby, 14 years ago,

41

her husband was diagnosed with an aggressive type of brain tumor. He died two years later when their son, Gilbert, was just 19 months old.

Andrea struggled through her husband's illness and eventual death. The emotional stress ravaged her body and unbalanced her hormones. She believes it was the tipping point that led to her developing a condition that she'll now be managing for the rest of her life — an autoimmune thyroid condition called Hashimoto's disease.

At first, Andrea's symptoms were mild, but she knew something was going on. Her waist was getting thicker. Her breasts were tender. Yet she ate a healthy diet and took great care of herself. Unfortunately, she couldn't get her physicians to pay attention to her thyroid because her lab markers were fine, and she was still functioning.

While her symptoms were mild, they continued to nag at her. Why was she feeling like this, she wondered. No one could give her answers. So she began to dig. After her own exhaustive research and meticulous investigation, she finally took her hunch to her doctor and asked, "Am I crazy, or is this Hashimoto's?"

The thing about Hashimoto's disease is that it's a "hidden" autoimmune condition. The symptoms aren't always as severe as in such illnesses as lupus or multiple sclerosis and, as a result, it often goes undiagnosed or improperly treated. After further testing, Andrea's doctor told her that she did indeed have Hashimoto's.

As soon as Andrea knew what was wrong with her, she began managing her condition. The first thing she did was to curb her desire to get better quickly. She became methodical about addressing all the underlying symptoms that exacerbated her condition.

She adjusted her diet to create what she called adrenal-gland support protocols. This low-glycemic diet meant that for the first nine months she ate absolutely no sugar. Her favorite foods, like raw honey and dried fruits, were out. She ate more foods rich in vitamin C, including supplements such as ashwagandha and rhodiola, to help build her adrenal reserve. She put herself on a strict bedtime schedule to get more sleep. Meanwhile she started working on her gut, because at the core of all autoimmune diseases, it's often assumed that there's a "leaky gut" involved. She ate probiotics and glutamine to heal her intestines and improve her reaction to food.

Andrea's recovery was methodical. She made changes slowly to not overwhelm herself. She paid attention to how she responded to each lifestyle change and waited until she was ready to tolerate a little more.

Today, Andrea credits her recovery to more than just protocols and diet. She believes her strengthened relationship with her body helped her attain a deeper state of healing. The routines she once struggled to maintain are now second nature. Regardless of how busy her day is, she's in bed by 9:30, which helps with the "brain fog" issues common in many people suffering from Hashimoto's. She eats a very low-glycemic diet with no sweeteners, except for Stevia. Once in a while she has a little coconut sugar or a single date or other dried fruit.

She feels strongly that nutrients are the key to basic health. A right diet is a place to start, but for some nutrients, we have to take supplements. These include probiotics, because our gut's microbiome is important to our immune health and mental health; Omega-3s, whether from good-quality fish or fish-oil supplements; B vitamins, for liver detoxification and brain health; and lastly, vitamin D3.

Andrea also constantly monitors her immune markers and her labs for thyroid markers and makes adjustments as needed. Last fall, for example, she discovered she had a particular hormone deficiency and was able to find a compounded hormone supplement to replace it.

As a single mom who runs a busy business, managing her health takes a great deal of time and energy. But because she has her illness under control, Andrea says, she feels great.

Now Andrea and her team apply the same approach she took to her own health to hundreds of clients around the world. Andrea's ability to uncover the root cause of health conditions allows her to help people where conventional professionals can't.

**Emma**
Emma was 12 years old when her parents brought her to see Andrea. She suffered from Crohn's disease and the first thing Andrea noticed was her diminutive size: very short and extremely skinny. Emma's personality came across as engaging and ambitious. This is common for people suffering from Crohn's disease, who are often overachievers. Emma's parents and her pediatric gastroenterologist were growing increasingly worried about her stature. She was already much smaller than her younger sister.

43

Andrea carefully studied Emma's diet and nutrition and suggested a few changes, along with various supplements. Within a few short months, Emma blossomed and began growing like a weed. Her mother was surprised and overjoyed that she needed a new pair of pants every few months. Andrea's recommended dietary regimen brought Emma completely into remission. She felt good, and her parents were thrilled.

Over the next few years, however, Emma became less disciplined with her diet, and her symptoms returned. She was starting high school and led a busy life: striving to get straight A's, performing in a school musical, and participating in various extracurricular activities. She soon discovered that she could not eat lunch while sitting on the floor with her friends, because that was too constrictive for her.

In a panic, Emma's parents brought her back to Andrea saying that their gastroenterologist wanted to put Emma on strong drugs and possibly remove part of her colon because of mucosal damage. After another examination, Andrea was convinced that it wasn't just mucosal damage; it was Emma's immune system attacking the mucus membranes of her colon. They just had to find out why it was happening again.

Emma tested positive for the bacteria dysbiosis. She also showed a high level of candida, likely related to eating foods with sugar — the hardest thing for Emma to stay away from.

Ultimately, Andrea agreed that Emma needed to go on the medication prescribed by her gastroenterologist. Her symptoms were too strong, and diet alone couldn't get her inflammation under control. At the same time, Andrea was adamant that Emma continue with the dietary and supplement protocol they initially put in place.

Today, Emma is doing well and is on her way to a full recovery. She and her parents are hoping she can soon stop taking her medication and manage her condition by diet alone. Andrea is also hopeful, saying, "When the inflammation is under control through diet and nutrient therapy, who's to say she can't go off the medication?"

**Healing Through Education**

Managing an autoimmune condition is a journey. At any time, a patient's immune system is vulnerable to overactivity. Almost anything can exacerbate an already-hyper immune system: stress, lack of sleep, travel, eating the wrong food, chemicals. Even when patients get to the point where they are asymptomatic, they still need to be vigilant.

Andrea believes the most important thing she does is teach people to listen to what's going on with their bodies. It's what's missing from our conventional medical model. Too often, people jump into treatment without understanding what's really happening. They just want the symptoms to go away.

Andrea and her team help patients develop a relationship with their body, to listen to signs and signals and ask what their body is trying to tell them. To constantly ask, "What's going on here?"

Andrea knows that everyone comes to the table with their own hang- ups about food, their condition, and their diagnosis. Taking these factors into consideration is part of the art of health counseling. In addition, Andrea prefers to work with her clients' physicians, so they have a team in place. When you're suffering from complicated health issues, it's powerful to have two or more people on your side, holding each other accountable to make sure nothing slips through the cracks. For Andrea and her team, that's what makes the difference.

---

*"It's my passion to help you to be the most viable collaborator in your own care. Ultimately this ability enables you to work with any physician to manage your signs and symptoms."*

*— Andrea (www.replenishpdx.com)*

# *Hashimoto's Disease Facts*

*"It is possible to fight and defeat the full spectrum of autoimmune diseases, from allergies and IBS to multiple sclerosis and Crohn's, without a cocktail of toxic treatments and medications."*
— *Mark Hyman, MD*

## What Is Hashimoto's Disease?

Hashimoto's disease is a condition in which your immune system attacks your thyroid, a small gland at the base of your neck below your Adam's apple.

## Warning Signs and Symptoms

You might not notice signs or symptoms of Hashimoto's disease at first, or notice a swelling at the front of your throat (goiter). Hashimoto's disease typically progresses slowly over years and causes chronic thyroid damage, leading to a drop in thyroid hormone levels in your blood.

- Fatigue and sluggishness
- Increased sensitivity to cold
- Constipation
- Pale, dry skin
- A puffy face
- Hoarse voice
- Unexplained weight gain — occurring infrequently and rarely exceeding 10 to 20 pounds, most of which is fluid
- Muscle aches, tenderness and stiffness, especially in your shoulders and hips
- Pain and stiffness in your joints and swelling in your knees or the small joints in your hands and feet
- Muscle weakness, especially in your lower extremities
- Excessive or prolonged menstrual bleeding (menorrhagia)
- Depression
- Tiredness for no apparent reason
- Dry skin
- Pale, puffy face
- Constipation
- Hoarse voice

**Statistics**
According to Hashimoto's Institute 1 in 5 Americans have hypothyroidism and only half of them know it. 97% of hypothyroidism cases are Hashimoto's Thyroiditis.

This disorder can affect anyone at any age but occurs most commonly in women who are over the age of 40. It may occur with increased frequency in those with a family history of thyroid diseases or with other autoimmune diseases, especially type 1 diabetes or adrenal insufficiency.

**Further Resources and Helpful Websites**
Lab Tests Online (labtestsonline.org)

# *Crohn's Disease Facts*

**What Is Crohn's Disease?**
Crohn's disease is a form of inflammatory bowel disease (IBD) and it usually affects the intestines, but may occur anywhere from the mouth to the end of the rectum (anus).

**Warning Signs and Symptoms**
Symptoms depend on what part of the digestive tract is involved and range from mild to severe. The main symptoms are:
- Crampy pain in the abdomen (belly area)
- Fever
- Fatigue
- Loss of appetite
- Feeling that you need to pass stools, even though your bowels are already empty
- Watery diarrhea, which may be bloody
- Weight loss

Other symptoms may include:
- Constipation
- Sores or swelling in the eyes
- Draining of pus, mucus, or stools from around the rectum or anus
- Joint pain and swelling
- Mouth ulcers
- Rectal bleeding and bloody stools

- Swollen gums
- Tender, red bumps (nodules) under the skin which may turn into skin ulcers

## Statistics

Nearly 1 in 200 Americans suffer with the debilitating and constant disruption of IBD. Crohn's can be found in both men and women; it may run in families, 20% of people diagnosed with the disease have a blood relative with some form of inflammatory bowel disease. It is usually diagnosed between the ages of 20 to 30, although people of all ages can suffer from Crohn's. People of Jewish heritage have a greater risk of developing the disease while people of African American heritage have less of a risk.

## Further Resources and Helpful Websites

U.S. National Library of Medicine
(www.ncbi.nlm.nih.gov/pubmedhealth)
Crohn's and Colitis Foundation of America (www.ccfa.org)
Just Crohn's (www.justcrohns.com)

# Part III

# Mood Disorders and Mental Illnesses

## 8

# From Suffering from Social Anxiety Disorder and Depression to Living a Fulfilled, Joyful Life

### Shayna's Secrets for Getting and Staying Off Prozac

*"Did you really want to die? No one commits suicide because they want to die. Then why do they do it? Because they want to stop the pain."*
*— Tiffanie DeBartolo*

*"Sometimes even to live is an act of courage."*
*— Seneca*

By the age of 12, Shayna had changed six schools. Her family moved often and, as a result, she endured constant life changes. What she longed for was a sense of stability.

Shayna had always lacked confidence and struggled with anxiety. When she was a baby, she suffered from separation anxiety and couldn't be left alone in a room. When she got older, it transformed into a social anxiety disorder. Having to start a new school and make new friends each year didn't help.

When Shayna was 12, her family moved from Arizona to Massachusetts. Once again she had to start at a new school. Seventh grade, as we all know, isn't the easiest age to make new friends, especially for someone suffering from social anxiety.

As Shayna's parents drove her to school, she sat in the back of the car sick to her stomach. All she wanted was to just go back home and lock herself in the house. So as soon as her parents dropped her off, Shayna would walk back home.

**A Tough Pill to Swallow**
Her parents hired a psychiatrist. They sent her to Boston Children's Hospital to help with her migraines and chronic stomachaches. They worked with the school to improve her attendance. Shayna had regular meetings with a guidance counselor.

However, having to spend a full day at school continued to feel horrible for her, so she was allowed to attend classes in the mornings and come back home in the afternoons. Shayna's psychologist officially diagnosed her with social anxiety disorder, separation anxiety, and depression. She was 12 years old, did not feel a sense of self-worth, and felt she was a burden to those around her. She felt hopeless and soon became suicidal.

Shayna was prescribed Prozac. By that time she felt so weak that she couldn't swallow her pills and had to take the liquid form of Prozac. It wasn't pleasant, and today, 15 years later, she can still recall the taste the liquid left in her mouth.

As hard as it was to take, the Prozac helped. Shayna was able to return to school, and by the end of the year, she went back to attending full school days. She felt much better and even began to make friends. In high school she experienced ups and downs. In some years, she would start out on top of things, and then she would start to feel depressed and anxious.

In Shayna's first year of college, her dad became seriously ill. She took on many of her dad's duties in the family business while juggling all her responsibilities as a first-year college student and worrying about his health. It was a terrifying, confusing, and highly stressful time in her life.

For the first time in her life, she began to gain weight, starting with 10 pounds when she was 18. She gained another 10 pounds the following year and 10 pounds more the year after that. By the time she was 22, she had gone from being underweight to 30 pounds overweight.

**Discovering an Alternative**
Shayna began researching prescription drugs and their effects on her body. Many members of her extended family had been on antidepressants for a long time, so she believed that she would always be taking them too. However, once she looked more closely at Prozac and its side effects, she began to question whether it was something she wanted to be taking forever.

She investigated alternatives to antidepressants and found Shaklee, a supplier of high-quality supplements. The first step of her healing journey was to learn about natural products and their effect on the body. She started taking a number of Shaklee supplements and began to feel better. The vitamins helped build up her immune system, and she found she was getting sick less often.

Encouraged, Shayna enrolled at a nutrition school, where she learned about the importance of a eating a healthier diet in addition to taking supplements. She altered her eating habits incrementally, such as adding more vegetables, drinking more water, and making spinach smoothies in the mornings. She also started exercising every day.

In a few short months, Shayna felt like her entire life changed. Her excess weight effortlessly vanished. Her skin cleared up. She felt more confident, happy, energized, and less anxious.

One side effect of Shayna's antidepressants was a constant feeling of numbness — a lack of emotion. She didn't want to feel "frozen" forever, so she decided to stop taking the pills and see what would happen. She was taking a lot of different mood-supportive vitamins and, under the guidance of her health counselor, she tapered off of Prozac.

Soon after, she discovered yoga, which further helped with her anxiety and depression. Being in the moment and focusing on her breathing helped her to slow down and stop being so worried. With her new-found flexibility came an increase in self-confidence.

She also began keeping a journal. Every night before going to bed, Shayna writes down five things that she is grateful for. It's made a huge difference in helping her concentrate on all the good things instead of focusing on the bad.

Today, Shayna is not taking any drugs. She's happy, less stressed, and less anxious. She left behind the girl who dreaded what each day would bring her. Despite this, Shayna says she still feels down at times. She is still shy and introverted. But she feels good knowing that she's able to take better care of herself. She's healthy, proud, and knows when she needs to slow down. And she keeps herself healthy with the right foods and lifestyle habits.

**Getting By with a Little Help**

For the things Shayna can't do alone, she's found others to assist her. She routinely sees a chiropractor. She works out with a personal trainer once a week. She gets a massage every few months. And she found a naturopathic doctor that she loves.

Over the years Shayna had seen many types of physicians, but seeing a naturopathic doctor was a completely different experience for her. On her first visit, the naturopath sat patiently with her for an hour and asked pointed questions to better understand what she was struggling with. They remained focused on Shayna and gave her as much time, support, encouragement, and help as she needed.

After learning that Shayna had gone through a severe case of mononucleosis in high school that damaged her immune system, her natruopath suggested that she take natural herbs to boost her immuninty. She helped Shayna manage her stress and anxiety naturally. She also helped bring her hormone levels into balance and improved her digestion.

In contrast, when Shayna asked her primary care doctor for help with her stomach issues, he sent her to a gastroenterologist, who in turn sent her to the pharmacy with a Metamucil prescription — which just made her feel even more bloated. She found that her conventional doctors did not really listen to her and were dismissive of her concerns about her health. They merely focused on eliminating symptoms — not treating the causes.

It's been almost 10 years since Shayna began on her road towards healing and recovery. She feels like this journey was a rebirth: starting out as a sad, hopeless, suicidal child and blossoming into the happy, vibrant, beautiful woman she is today.

---

*"Forget unhealthy diets, harmful medications, and emotional roller coasters. Heal depression naturally, and find your true path to happiness"*

— *Shayna (www.shaynamahoney.com)*

# *Social Anxiety Disorder Facts*

*"**Anxiety** is an enormously crippling problem. Most people in this country suffer with it and do nothing, or they resort to drugs. Drugs do help, but it is obvious that they are no more than Band-Aids...*

***Depression** is expected to be the second leading cause of disability for people of all ages by 2020, so this is an issue that impacts many, many people."*
— *Dr. Joseph Mercola*

---

## What Is Social Anxiety Disorder?
Social anxiety disorder is a disorder in which a person has an excessive and unreasonable fear of social situations.

## Warning Signs and Symptoms
Emotional and behavioral symptoms of social anxiety disorder can include:

- Fear of situations in which you may be judged
- Worrying about embarrassing or humiliating yourself
- Concern that you'll offend someone
- Intense fear of interacting or talking with strangers
- Fear that others will notice that you look anxious
- Fear of physical symptoms that may cause you embarrassment, such as blushing, sweating, trembling or having a shaky voice
- Avoiding doing things or speaking to people out of fear of embarrassment
- Avoiding situations where you might be the center of attention
- Having anxiety in anticipation of a feared activity or event
- Spending time after a social situation analyzing your performance and identifying flaws in your interactions
- Expecting the worst possible consequences from a negative experience during a social situation

Physical signs and symptoms can sometimes accompany social anxiety disorder and may include:

- Fast heartbeat
- Upset stomach or nausea
- Trouble catching your breath
- Dizziness or lightheadedness

- Confusion or feeling "out of body"
- Diarrhea
- Muscle tension
- Blushing
- Profuse sweating
- Trembling
- Headaches

Common, everyday experiences that may be hard to endure when you have social anxiety disorder include, for example:
- Using a public restroom
- Interacting with strangers
- Eating in front of others
- Making eye contact
- Initiating conversations
- Dating
- Attending parties or social gatherings
- Missing work or school
- Entering a room in which people are already seated
- Returning items to a store

**Anxiety and Depression**
It's not uncommon for someone with an anxiety disorder to also suffer from depression, or vice versa. Nearly one-half of those diagnosed with depression are also diagnosed with an anxiety disorder.

**Causes**
Like many other mental health conditions, social anxiety disorder likely arises from a complex interaction of environment and genes. Possible causes include:
- Inherited traits. Anxiety disorders tend to run in families.
- Brain structure. A structure in the brain called the amygdala may play a role in controlling the fear response.
- Environment. Social anxiety disorder may be a learned behavior. That is, you may develop the condition after witnessing the anxious behavior of others.

**Statistics**
Anxiety disorders are the most common mental illness in the U.S., affecting 40 million adults in the United States age 18 and older (18% of the U.S. population). About 15 million (6.8%) American adults have

social anxiety disorder.
- Typical age of onset: 13 years old
- 36 percent of people with social anxiety disorder report symptoms for 10 or more years before seeking help
- Equally common among men and women, typically beginning around age 13
- According to a 2007 ADAA survey, 36% of people with social anxiety disorder report experiencing symptoms for 10 or more years before seeking help

**Further Resources and Helpful Websites**
Anxiety and Depression Association of America, ADAA (www.adaa.org)
WebMD (www.webmd.com)

# 9
# *Healing Bipolar Disorder*
# *and Depression Without Drugs*

*"My mother called me 'Crazy Gracie' as a child, a term of endearment for my energetic creativity. I was not diagnosed as bipolar until 1993, when a therapist noticed manic highs between my life-long bouts of depression. After refusing lithium due to its side effects, I was placed on an antidepressant. Life seemed easier, less chaotic. A year later breast cysts and tumors appeared rapidly and I had surgery twice in twelve months. Each time growths were cut out, more would develop. Doctors said all they could do was monitor the lumps until one proved malignant. Waiting for cancer didn't sound like a great plan, so I went searching for other options."*
*— From "Who's Crazy Here?" by Gracelyn Guyol*

Gracelyn grew up on a working farm in Hillsdale, Michigan. In her late teens, she began to experience occasional periods of depression. She was too young and inexperienced to know exactly what was going on.

Her depressions remained mild and infrequent until her late 30s. Then things began to change. She was running a PR agency, beginning a new marriage, mothering a teenager, and building a new home. And she was under a lot of stress. Her depressions occurred more frequently and were sometimes immobilizing.

Gracelyn's lifelong bouts of depression were finally diagnosed as bipolar disorder. She was prescribed a routine antidepressant. Within a year, she developed a rapid growth of breast cysts and tumors. She underwent two difficult surgeries, altering the course of her entire life.

The drug that triggered breast cyst and tumor growth was Wellbutrin. Her psychiatrist said that research showed an increase in mammary tumors in mice, but the findings were deemed inconclusive because the mice were given 9,000 times what a human would take by weight.

When Gracelyn had the last tumor biopsied, she asked her doctors if they had noticed whether women on antidepressants developed breast cancer more frequently. She was told they hadn't looked at that, but they had casually observed these women had more breast discharge, so they knew the drugs affected breast tissue.

**Gracelyn's Journey**

Gracelyn felt betrayed by the American Medical Association and medical profession — that the pills that were supposed to help relieve her depression and mania were actually triggering the rapid growth of breast cysts and tumors. Her tumors were life threatening, yet her psychiatrists had never mentioned the risks associated with her medication. This realization was one of the hardest moments in Gracelyn's life. It was also life altering and awakening. It marked the beginning of Gracelyn's journey towards finding safer and more effective ways to feel better and, eventually, heal.

The journey led her to discover dozens of safer, less expensive, holistic options that actually restore mental balance. Under the direction of a naturopathic doctor, Gracelyn took a holistic approach to stop the rapid growths of the malignant cells in her body. Together they focused on systematically eliminating substances that might cause cells to mutate. They dramatically changed Gracelyn's diet, added therapeutic levels of vitamins, minerals, and other nutrients, and systematically worked to reduce contact with chemicals or toxins that might make cells mutate.

These same steps were part of the process necessary to clear toxins from her body, provide essential nutrients to her brain cells, and help restore mental balance. Cyst growth soon halted, but a new benign breast tumor appeared in 1998. The only chemical Gracelyn still knowingly took was the antidepressant. She tapered off the antidepressant pills to see what would happen. Within eight weeks, her latest tumor disappeared and all growths stopped.

Gracelyn was thrilled with her success. However, she also knew that she had to figure out how to help her brain function without drugs as she realized that mood swings were going to get worse with age. Refusing all psychiatric medications, she spent two years seeking holistic solutions that ended her bipolar symptoms.

Instead of attempting to simply manage her illness with expensive, patented, dangerous drugs, Gracelyn halt symptoms using natural supplements and therapies that, in addition, brought "side benefits" of improved overall health. Had Gacelyn not been proactive, she would no doubt have had one of her tumors become malignant. She side-stepped breast cancer.

Remarkably, anyone diagnosed or undiagnosed with bipolar, can get better through holistic steps. There are laboratory tests, available for two decades, that help identify the nutrient deficits. Once someone is tested, they can easily compensate for these nutrient deficiencies using natural substances.

Not only is this approach easier, but it's also more effective and less harmful to the patient. It's also substantially less expensive compared to conventional treatment. While supplements cost between $60 and $150 per month, co-pay costs of psychiatric medications can easily cost upwards of $200 per month. Yet conventionally trained doctors are taught nothing about inexpensive, holistic treatments due to decades of pharmaceutical-industry-funded American Medical Association conferences, university research, and the influence of government legislators.

The amount of money that Gracelyn spent out of pocket to end her bipolar symptoms was $3,000. It was all that was needed for her to get well within shortest amount of time and without risking her health. Gracelyn recovered in the following four steps that she developed:

1. Find an alternative medical practitioner to guide you.
2. Systematize your diet.
   - Eat a nutrient-dense diet.
   - Eat three small meals and two snacks per day to keep blood sugar and moods stable.
   - Eliminate hydrogenated and trans-fats from your diet that block the use of good fats.
   - Take daily supplements containing 3–5 grams per day of essential Omega-3 fish oil.
   - Take high-quality vitamins and minerals to ensure you're getting nutrients required for healthy brain functions. Consider those developed specifically for bipolar disorder.
3. Alter your daily routine.
   - Get 30–45 minutes of daily exercise to infuse your brain with oxygen.
   - Reduce stress.
   - Get eight hours of sleep every night.
4. Establish the reasons and resolve the causes
   - Test for genetic errors.
   - Test for thyroid and other hormone imbalances.
   - Test for vitamin, mineral, and amino acid imbalances, making adjustments as needed.

- When you are sufficiently stable, ask your practitioner to direct you how to safely taper off psychiatric drugs that cause many symptoms.
- Test gut flora and replenish beneficial bacteria for better absorption and use of nutrients.
- Test for and address food allergies and sensitivities that often cause "brain allergies" contributing to symptoms.
- If candida overgrowth is present, follow lowering diet and biological solutions.
- Test for genetic metal metabolism errors (Metallothionein profile through www.greatplainslaboratory.com) or for heavy metals overload and begin detoxification.
- Begin therapy to help with any past emotional trauma.

Today, Gracelyn is 67 and in a great physical shape. She weighs the same as she did in high school and feels vibrant and energetic. She takes no prescription medications. She plays tennis and does yoga a few times a week. She's generally positive, maintains her sense of humor, and feels her moods stay within normal fluctuations.

In addition to ending the tumors and bipolar symptoms, she freed herself of arthritis and avoided Type 2 diabetes, which is rampant in her family. Gracelyn used to wonder with envy how other people's lives seemed so easy. Just keeping herself organized required a tremendous amount of energy.

Now, without her bipolar mood swings, she feels like a giant boulder has been lifted off her shoulders. Suddenly, everything — work, study, relationships, hobbies — seems simple. Her life has become balanced.

---

*"You are in charge of rebuilding your mental health. An experienced holistic practitioner can outline a plan and provide guidance. You'll notice a slight increase in energy, more focus and calm, the ability to make decisions easier, less chaos in your life, and perhaps more laughter. This is the road to recovery. It always has a few potholes but it is the most promising route."*

*— Gracelyn (www.crazyrecovery.com)*

# *Bipolar Disorder Facts*

*"There's no sure way to prevent bipolar disorder. However, getting treatment at the earliest sign of a mental health disorder can help prevent bipolar disorder or other mental health conditions from worsening."*
— *Mayo Clinic*

## What Is Bipolar Disorder?

Bipolar disorder is a serious mental illness that is characterized by extreme changes in mood, from mania to depression. It can lead to risky behavior, damaged relationships and careers, and even suicidal tendencies if it's not treated.

## Causes

Bipolar disorder affects men and women equally. Western medicine maintains that the exact cause is not known, although it's well established that bipolar occurs more often in relatives of people with bipolar disorder. Holistic practitioners, however, have identified numerous common causes that, once addressed, bring about recovery. For example, the work of Dr. William Walsh has shown that episodes of extreme happiness and high activity or energy (mania) are commonly caused by elevated copper brought on by inherited errors. Any of the following may trigger a manic episode:

- Stress
- Severe emotional trauma, such as incest, rape, horrific accidents, or battle experiences
- Childbirth
- Medicines such as antidepressants or steroids
- Periods of not being able to sleep (insomnia)
- Recreational drug use

Psychiatrists are taught that mood swings from mania to depression always go together in bipolar disorder. Yet holistic practitioners find the causes of bipolar depression are distinct from those of mania. Substances and conditions causing depression include:

- Junk food diet with high transfat content
- Hypothyroidism or other hormone imbalances
- Essential fatty acid deficiencies
- Low Vitamin D levels
- Prescription drugs

61

## Warning Signs and Symptoms

The manic phase may last from days to months. It can include these symptoms:

- Easily distracted
- Little need for sleep
- Poor judgment
- Poor temper control
- Reckless behavior and lack of self-control such as drinking, drug use, sex with many partners, spending sprees
- Very irritable mood, such as racing thoughts, talking a lot, false beliefs about self or abilities
- Very involved in activities
- The depressive episode may include these symptoms:
- Daily low mood or sadness
- Difficulty concentrating, remembering, or making decisions
- Eating problems such as loss of appetite and weight loss, or overeating and weight gain
- Fatigue or lack of energy
- Feeling worthless, hopeless, or guilty

## Statistics

Bipolar disorder affects approximately 5.7 million adult Americans, or about 2.6% of the U.S. population age 18 and older every year. (National Institute of Mental Health)

The median age of onset for bipolar disorder is 25 years (National Institute of Mental Health), although the illness can start in early childhood or as late as the 40's and 50's. An equal number of men and women develop bipolar illness and it is found in all ages, races, ethnic groups and social classes. More than two-thirds of people with bipolar disorder have at least one close relative with the illness or with unipolar major depression, indicating the disease has a heritable component. (National Institute of Mental Health)

## Women and Bipolar Disorder

Although bipolar disorder is equally common in women and men, research indicates that approximately three times as many women as men experience rapid cycling. (Journal of Clinical Psychiatry, 58, 1995 [Suppl.15]) Other research findings indicate that women with bipolar disorder may have more depressive episodes and more mixed episodes than do men with the illness. (Journal of Clinical Psychiatry, 58, 1995 [Suppl.15])

## Economic Factors

Bipolar disorder is the sixth leading cause of disability in the world. (World Health Organization)

## Suicide and Bipolar Disorder

Bipolar disorder results in 9.2 years reduction in expected life span, and as many as one in five patients with bipolar disorder completes suicide. (National Institute of Mental Health)

## Children and Adolescents

Bipolar disorder is more likely to affect the children of parents who have the disorder. When one parent has bipolar disorder, the risk to each child is 15 to 30%. When both parents have bipolar disorder, the risk increases to 50 to 75%. (National Institute of Mental Health)

Bipolar Disorder may be at least as common among youth as among adults. In a recent NIMH study, one percent of adolescents ages 14 to 18 were found to have met criteria for bipolar disorder or cyclothymia in their lifetime. (National Institute of Mental Health) Some 20% of adolescents with major depression develop bipolar disorder within five years of the onset of depression. (Birmaher, B., "Childhood and Adolescent Depression: A Review of the Past 10 Years." Part I, 1995)

Up to one-third of the 3.4 million children and adolescents with depression in the United States may actually be experiencing the early onset of bipolar disorder. (American Academy of Child and Adolescent Psychiatry, 1997)

When manic, children and adolescents, in contrast to adults, are more likely to be irritable and prone to destructive outbursts than to be elated or euphoric. When depressed, there may be many physical complaints such as headaches, and stomachaches or tiredness; poor performance in school, irritability, social isolation, and extreme sensitivity to rejection or failure. (National Institute of Mental Health).

## Why New Approach is Needed

- 50% of patients do not respond to psychiatric medications at all. Of those who benefit, half go off due to side effects:
- 30-60 lb. weight gain
- 58% sexual dysfunction (SSRIs)
- 40% develop tics (from antipsychotics), drowsiness, feeling "drugged", insomnia, depression and suicidality

**Where To Find The New Approach Method:**
Gracelyn Guyol Author, Producer, TV series "Restoring Health Holistically"
Most addiction programs achieve long-term abstinence of 310%. The approach Gracelyn recommends (which actually *treats the physical causes of addiction*) enjoys a 60-74% success rate. Even children with autism, the most complex disorder, can often recover.

***"Healing Depression & Bipolar Disorder Without Drugs"*** (2006) *by Gracelyn Guyol*
A road map that gives science-based explanations for healing.

***"Who's Crazy Here?"*** *(2010) by Gracelyn Guyol*
Offers brief instructions and nondrug Steps to Recovery for nine major mental disorders. Gracelyn is now working on a book about preventing Alzheimers (anyone who has been depressed for years has a 30% higher risk of it).

**More on the subject:**
"The Mood Cure" by Julia Ross "Nutrient Power" by Dr. William Walsh

**Further Resources and Helpful Websites**
U.S. National Library of Medicine: PubMed health
(www.ncbi.nlm.nih.gov/pubmedhealth)
Depression and Bipolar Support Alliance (www.dbsalliance.org)

# 10
# Feeling Tapped Out

*Overcoming anxiety and depression with EFT*

*"People tend to dwell more on negative things than on good things. So the mind then becomes obsessed with negative things, with judgments, guilt and anxiety produced by thoughts about the future and so on."*
— *Eckhart Tolle*

Tina was thrilled to learn that her husband had landed his dream job after months of being out of work. The position was a perfect fit for him. They could finally stop worrying about bills. The only downside was that the job was 500 miles away.

Tina chose to stay behind. Their kids had grown and left for college, so she would be left alone in the house. She feared it would get lonely, but Tina was also excited at the prospect of having a little more freedom. She knew her life had become increasingly more managed by others over the course of her adult life. She just didn't know by how much.

Tina's husband was an engineer. He was as meticulous and exacting at home as he was at work. Tina was often on edge, paying extra attention to keeping things in a precise order. The bed had to be made a certain way each morning. Dinner had to be ready at seven each night. Household items had to be put in particular places.

Suddenly, Tina had the freedom to do as she pleased. If she didn't want to make the bed, it could stay rumpled all day. She could eat dinner at ten-o'clock if she chose. She no longer had to consider anyone in making plans for the day. And as strange as it felt at the beginning, the strangeness didn't last. It soon felt comfortable and easy. After two years of living alone, Tina got used to it.

When her husband accepted a new job near their house and moved back home, Tina found the transition to be hard. They had to learn to live together again. Of course she loved her husband dearly. She appreciated his dedication in taking care of her and their kids all those years. But now the way of life she had gotten used to was in upheaval. Having to do things she wasn't used to anymore made her feel anxious and, consequently, angry. Mostly angry at herself for being anxious. Tina felt

65

stuck and unable to get a handle on her emotions. She became further frustrated with herself. She soon began noticing physical symptoms of anxiety and fatigue.

At this point, Tina was desperate. She tried her best to "hang in there," while actively looking for help. One morning she came across an article about Emotional Freedom Technique (EFT) on Dr. Mercola's website (see Resources, below). It's a healing technique that connects the Chinese meridian system with tapping on various body parts with your fingers.

At first glance Tina thought, "What crazy stuff! People just tap on themselves and feel better?" But she didn't have a better solution — and she certainly had nothing to lose — so she decided to keep an open mind. She printed out an online manual to sift through on the beach the following weekend. She began to go through the mechanics of tapping, and the effects were dramatic. Tina quickly saw EFT as a powerful, effective technique for getting at suppressed feelings. It wasn't long before she was tapping into her own negative emotions.

The primary feeling that emerged for Tina was anger. Tapping helped her discover that the root of her anxiety was her body asking: "Can we deal with this feeling?" She had been burying her negative feelings for so long that they manifested into physical symptoms — the only way her body knew how to communicate with her.

After three rounds of tapping, five minutes each, her anger almost disappeared and she felt her energy shift. In a matter of weeks, Tina was able to relieve all of the symptoms she had been suffering from. Through tapping, she was finally able to get at what she was feeling. And she let it all out. Now, almost seven years later, Tina has become a major EFT advocate and a proud practitioner using this powerful tool to help others who feel depressed, tired, anxious, or sad.

---

*"If you experience emotions that you wish to change — EFT is a self-help tool you can use any time, and not have to wait for a therapy appointment."*
— *Tina (www.medicinemyway.us)*

# *General Anxiety Facts*

*"Life experience is not about what happened to you. It's really about the meaning you make about what happened to you."*
*— NLP paradigm*

## What Is Anxiety?
Anxiety is an unpleasant state of inner turmoil, often accompanied by nervous behavior, such as pacing back and forth, somatic complaints, and rumination. Anxiety disorders develop from a complex set of risk factors, including genetics, brain chemistry, personality, and life events.

## Warning Signs and Symptoms
Depending on the type of anxiety disorder, general symptoms include:
- Feelings of panic, fear, and uneasiness
- Problems sleeping
- Cold or sweaty hands and/or feet
- Shortness of breath
- Heart palpitations
- An inability to be still and calm
- Dry mouth
- Numbness or tingling in the hands or feet
- Nausea
- Muscle tension
- Dizziness

## Generalized Anxiety Disorder (GAD)
GAD Symptoms:
People with generalized anxiety disorder experience constant, chronic, and unsubstantiated worry, often about health, family, money, or work. This worrying disrupts social activities and interferes with work, school, or family.

Physical symptoms of GAD include the following:
- Muscle tension
- Fatigue
- Restlessness
- Difficulty sleeping
- Irritability

- Edginess
- Gastrointestinal discomfort or diarrhea

**Statistics**

Anxiety disorders are the most common mental illnesses in the U.S., affecting 40 million adults (18 percent of U.S. population). GAD affects million adults, or 3.1 percent of the U.S. population, in any given year. Women are twice as likely to be affected.

**Further Resources and Helpful Websites**

Anxiety and Depression Association of America (www.adaa.org)

## *EFT – Emotional Freedom Technique Facts*

**What is EFT?**

Emotional Freedom Technique (EFT) is a form of counseling intervention that draws on various theories of alternative medicine including acupuncture, neurolinguistic programming (NLP), energy medicine, and Thought Field Therapy (TFT). It is best known through Gary Craig's *EFT Handbook*, published in the late 1990s.

One of EFT's most fascinating features is that your "story" becomes not as important as the accompanying feeling (sadness, guilt, shame, resentment, etc.). EFT doesn't change your story. Rather, it helps to change your feelings and the meaning you make of your story.

**Further Resources and Helpful Websites**

www.eft.mercola.com
www.thetappingsolution.com
www.doctoroz.com/videos/webexclusivetappingtechnique

# Part IV

# Oncological Diseases

## 11

## *Curing the Incurable and Restoring Health Holistically*

*By Greg Culver*

*"Eighty-five percent of all disease is a lifestyle choice."*
— *Dr. Brian Clement, Hippocrates Health Institute*

*"Have an open mind and take in what you are ready to take in."*
— *Dr. Anne-Marie Clement, Hippocrates Health Institute*

---

In 2008, Jackie went through a breast cancer ordeal. Regrettably, she didn't learn about the Hippocrates Life Transformation Program until years later. Researching had become one of the Jackie's weapons against the disease. Reading *The China Study* by T. Colin Campbell helped her learn about the vital link between cancer and lifestyle.

She was an optometrist, and because her practice was a short walk from a coffee shop, she survived on coffee and sugar while working sixty- hour weeks. She was attached to computers and her cell phone, worked under fluorescent lighting with little sun and fresh air, breathed toxins from a newly renovated office, and ate meat and dairy three times a day — often processed, usually microwaved.

After rejecting chemotherapy and radiation prescribed for her Stage 2, estrogen-positive breast cancer, Jackie adopted a plant-based lifestyle. Moreover, she closed her practice and reopened as a wellness center so she could access complimentary medicine and unplug for a while.

At that time, she didn't understand the difference between raw vegan and a "living foods" diet. She substituted processed sugars for agave, maple syrup, honey, and other "natural sweeteners." As a result, silently, her sugar addiction wreaked havoc on her bones.

### A SAD Way of Life
Over the next four years, as Jackie returned to her full-time practice, she slipped back into her old standard American diet ("SAD"), full of processed sugars. Unsurprisingly, she gained 50 pounds, experienced hot flashes, and had an increase in overall inflammation. She thought it was old age when her back began to hurt. She was 49.

Unbearable sciatic nerve pain brought her to her chiropractor and good friend, Dr. Chris Deveau. When the treatments did not relieve the pain, he performed an x-ray and MRI and discovered unusual compression fractures. On April 15th, 2014, Jackie was diagnosed with Stage 4 metastatic cancer.

Jackie didn't have health insurance and was in pain. Unable to walk, dress herself, or care for her family, she had to stop working. The weather in Connecticut was freezing, which worsened her sciatic pain. Six days following her diagnosis, with the support of her advanced practice registered nurse, Rebecca Murray, and Dr. Deveau, Jackie arrived at Hippocrates West Palm Beach campus.

She was barely able to walk.

Jackie was given a unique test called CyberScan. Dr. Paul, the doctor on staff, recommended IV injections and oxygen therapies to boost her immune system.

While at Hippocrates, Jackie enjoyed "living foods" for the first time. She was instructed not to eat sugar — not even fruit. She was put on an anti-inflammatory diet and other treatments. Warm mineral pools gave her relief and made her feel weightless. She participated in the Aqua-Motion physical therapy program. However, what Jackie felt helped most was the love and dedication of the Hippocrates staff, who helped her believe that she could reclaim her health. In three weeks, she lost 26 pounds and felt her pain subside.

**Back to Health**
Jackie underwent a significant improvement supported by the program. But despite her gains, much of her body remained in very serious condition. Cancer eroded three bones and had invaded her hips, neck, and ribs. She required surgery to stabilize her spine. So during an eight-hour procedure, her orthopedic surgeon fused six vertebrae together, and in the process, saved her ability to use her legs.

Jackie's husband, Greg, was supportive throughout her treatment. He grew sprouts and wheatgrass and brought it to Jackie daily to help her maintain the anti-inflammatory diet she learned at Hippocrates.

Having lost nearly 50 pounds at this point, Jackie healed very quickly and did not require any pain medication, thanks to Lisa Zaccheo, her hypnotherapist, and the integrative team at Backus Hospital. Nevertheless, her oncologists were anxious to have her undergo radiation and medication to treat her tumor.

It didn't inspire confidence in Jackie that ice cream was being served near the entry hall to the radiology department. The doctors didn't seem to recognize the relationship between diet and the illness they were treating. Jackie wished she could give them each a copy of *The China Study*.

She opted for a second opinion with an integrative, nutritional oncologist from Yale, Dr. Barry Boyd. In August, a PET scan revealed that the cancer was not advancing. There were no cancer cells in her lumbar spine! Dr. Barry Boyd recognized that the Hippocrates diet was naturally regulating Jackie's estrogen. Cancer markers were reduced, as well as glucose cholesterol and blood pressure.

Jackie was taking no medication and had tremendous energy for someone two months post-op with a diagnosis of incurable Stage 4 metastatic cancer.

**Sprouting a New Business**
Greg and Jackie wanted to share their journey with their community so they invited Dr. Clement, from the Hippocrates Health Institute, to speak in Mystic, Connecticut. Nearly 500 people attended the "Survive or Thrive" event.

This led Jackie and Greg to launch a new business, Sprout It Out, and the Mini Hippocrates Immersion Program, where they teach others how and why to enjoy living foods. They know firsthand that it's easier to embrace change when someone is facing a life-threatening illness. For those seeking illness prevention or weight loss, it may be harder to initiate change or justify taking time away from work. So Jackie and Greg help people make the transition to the Hippocrates way of living with a taste of their program.

---

*"The tumors are just 'warning' signs of the condition the body is in. The true healing comes from a change in diet, a change in thinking, and a change in how one lives. This was a paradigm shift for our entire family and the best thing we ever did."*

— Jackie (www.jackieshealthblog.blogspot.com)

# *Breast Cancer Facts*

*When detected and treated early, cancer can often be stopped. That said, cancer is a leading cause of death and disability around the world.*
*— Harvard Health Publications, Harvard Medical School*

## What Is Breast cancer?
Breast cancer is a malignant tumor that starts in the cells of the breast.

## What Is Metastatic Cancer?
Metastatic cancer is cancer that has spread from the place where it first started to another place in the body.

## Warning Signs and Symptoms of Breast Cancer
The most common symptom of breast cancer is a new lump or mass. A lump that is painless, hard, and has uneven edges is more likely to be cancer, but some cancers are tender, soft, and rounded or even painful.

Other symptoms of breast cancer include the following:
- Swelling of all or part of the breast
- Skin irritation or dimpling
- Breast pain
- Nipple pain or the nipple turning inward
- Redness, scaliness, or thickening of the nipple or breast skin
- A nipple discharge other than breast milk

## Warning Signs and Symptoms of Metastatic Cancer
Some people with metastatic tumors do not have symptoms and their metastases are found by x-rays or other tests. When symptoms of metastatic cancer occur, the type and frequency of the symptoms will depend on the size and location of the metastasis.

## Statistics for Breast Cancer
Breast cancer is the most common cancer among American women, except for skin cancers. About 1 in 8 (12%) women in the US will develop invasive breast cancer during their lifetime. The American Cancer Society's estimates for breast cancer in the United States for 2014 are:
- About 232,670 new cases of invasive breast cancer will be diagnosed in women

- About 62,570 new cases of carcinoma in situ (CIS) will be diagnosed (CIS is non-invasive and is the earliest form of breast cancer)
- About 40,000 women will die from breast cancer

Number of New Cases and Deaths per 100,000: The number of new cases of breast cancer was 124.6 per 100,000 women per year. The number of deaths was 22.2 per 100,000 women per year. These rates are age-adjusted and based on 2007-2011 cases and deaths.

Lifetime Risk of Developing Cancer: Approximately 12.3 percent of women will be diagnosed with breast cancer at some point during their lifetime, based on 2009-2011 data.

Prevalence of this cancer: In 2011, there were an estimated 2,899,726 women living with breast cancer in the United States.

**Statistics for Metastatic Cancer**
New Cases: The number of new cases each year of metastatic breast cancer is unknown but consists of those initially diagnosed stage IV and those who had early stage breast cancer and have a metastatic recurrence:
- Approximately 6–10% of new breast cancer cases are initially Stage IV or metastatic
- This is sometimes called "de novo" metastatic disease, meaning from the beginning
- It is estimated that 20–30% of all breast cancer cases will become metastatic

Living with MBC: The number of people living with metastatic breast cancer in the US is estimated to be over 155,000, but no statistics are currently collected.

Median Survival: Median survival after a metastatic breast cancer diagnosis is three years. Median survival in 1970 was 18 months.

Deaths in the U.S.: Despite the decrease in cancer mortality rates since 1990, the actual number of Americans losing their battle with the disease has hovered around 40,000 each year since at least the year 2000. (American Cancer Society statistics 2000–2011)
- Breast cancer is the most common cancer in women worldwide. It is also the principal cause of death from cancer among women globally. (World Health Organization)

- Race: Compared to white women, African-American women are diagnosed at a higher rate under age 40 and are more likely to die from breast cancer at every age.
- Young Women: Breast cancer is the number one cause of cancer death in young women under age 50. Although breast cancer is often described as a "disease of aging," 16% of the breast cancer deaths in 2012 were in this age group.
- Men: Men do get breast cancer and represent approximately 1% of the new cases and deaths from breast cancer in the US.

**Further Resources and Helpful Websites**
National Cancer Institute at the National Institute of Health (http://www.cancer.gov)
American Cancer Society (http://www.cancer.org)
Metastatic Breast Cancer Network (http://mbcn.org)
"Cancer metastasis as a therapeutic target" European Journal of Cancer 46 (2010) 1177-1180. Steeg, Patricia and Sleeman, Jonathan.

# 12
# Becoming a Warrior for His Health

*"Cancer is a word, not a sentence."*
— *John Diamond*

---

They were seated in their family doctor's office, waiting. Finally the doctor came in. He looked at Jim and said, "You have stage four non-Hodgkin's lymphoma."

Stage. Four. Cancer.

Suzanne repeated the doctor's words in her head, trying to understand what she'd just heard.

Stage. Four. Cancer.

She knew that from that point on, their lives would never be the same.

**Developing Symptoms**
Jim and Suzanne had always been interested in fitness and wellness. They met at a health club, where they both worked as weightlifting instructors.

To support and maintain their health throughout their busy and stressful daily routines, they regularly saw a naturopathic doctor. When he suggested they undergo a 28-day juice cleanse, they were gladly on board. After 14 days, Jim crashed. He felt terrible, and they assumed it was because he didn't incorporate the recommended lifestyle changes into his stressful daily routine. He lost about 10 pounds, as expected, but unlike Suzanne, he didn't put any weight back on after the cleanse was over. He also began experiencing digestive problems and had difficulty breathing while sleeping. And despite his weight loss, he was oddly bloated. He couldn't button his pants.

Uncertain how to get back to normal, Jim went to see his chiropractor. While he was being adjusted, Jim mentioned his digestive issues. Following a quick examination, his chiropractor exclaimed, "Oh my gosh, Jim. That's your spleen! That's really enlarged, you have to get to a doctor."

The next day he and Suzanne went to see their family doctor and were informed of Jim's stage four non-Hodgkin's lymphoma. At this point, he had been having noticeable symptoms for two months. The tumor in his spleen was football size. The cancer had spread to his abdominal lymph node — and his bone narrow. The pressure of the tumor against his other organs explained why he was having trouble digesting his food, why he had difficulty breathing.

He was referred to an oncologist, who sent him to the Memorial Sloan Kettering Cancer Center in New York City, routinely ranked the best in the nation for cancer care.

He and Suzanne were asked if they wanted to have kids. His physicians suggested he visit a sperm bank before his treatments, because, most probably, he wouldn't be able to have children afterwards. This was the day before his treatments were scheduled to begin. Jim felt awfully sick. He and Suzanne had talked about having children, but now they just wanted him to survive. They said no.

Jim was 38 years old. His many years of eating well and disciplined workouts added to the shock for him and everyone who knew him.

**Environmental and Emotional Causes**
According to the National Institutes of Health, only five to ten percent of all cancer cases can be attributed to genetic defects, whereas the remaining 90 to 95 percent have their roots in the environment and lifestyle: obesity, stress, environmental toxins, radiation, and viruses.

Lymphoma is an environmental cancer, and this fact led to Jim looking back at his life and questioning where he went "wrong." Was he to blame for his illness? When he was younger, he worked as a church groundskeeper. He remembered eating a sandwich while spreading weed killer. Could that have caused his cancer?

Suzanne helped him walk through his childhood, questioning some emotional events that played a big role in shaping his life. When Jim was a baby, his mother turned him over to her parents to raise him. This led to a great deal of resentment and feelings of rejection. There were a lot of unresolved issues festering inside of him, including anger directed toward his mom.

## Conventional Treatment and Unconventional Questions

At Sloan Kettering, Jim was diagnosed with two types of lymphoma: low-growing, low-grade and an aggressive grade. It was a rare diagnosis for someone as young as Jim. His doctors refused to even discuss the possibility of remission. Instead, they focused on keeping him comfortable and hoped that science would overcome his disease.

Since his cancer had spread, he wouldn't have surgery. He was treated with chemotherapy, along with a new drug, Rituxan, which had just received FDA approval a few months prior to Jim's diagnosis. Unlike standard chemotherapy drugs, which kill both cancerous and healthy cells, Rituxan is a "smart" drug, targeting only cancer cells.

Jim and Suzanne's days were filled with doctor's appointments, treatments, numerous tests, and constant fear. Suzanne felt powerless and wished there were more she could do to help. She kept asking Jim's doctors, "What can we do differently at home?" "How can we transform our lifestyles to help fight this cancer?" "Are there certain diets Jim should be eating?" and "Are there supplements he should be taking?"

The response was always basically the same: "No, just go live your life. Eat what you like, enjoy yourself, and don't bother with supplements."

Suzanne soon realized that they would have to figure out Jim's prevention strategies on their own. She started with the things that they had control over: What Jim drinks. What he eats. What he thinks. How he moves.

## Creating the Plan

Jim was diagnosed in 1999, when the Internet wasn't anything like it is now. Google wasn't yet a verb. Nonetheless, Suzanne found several chat-rooms where she met others who were struggling with lymphoma, and she was able to learn from their experiences.

While Suzanne did the research, reading and reaching out to people, constantly worrying, Jim was able to keep his head up and stay positive while focusing on healing. When Suzanne would find something interesting, she would let Jim know about it.

Suzanne pored through books about beating cancer and learned about the importance of staying away from sugar. It was a theory that made perfect sense to her. And it raised the question of why Jim's doctors wouldn't tell him that. Why weren't there billboards stating that to battle cancer you have to stay away from sugar, she wondered.

Eventually, Suzanne and Jim came up with their own plan of action.

While the doctors did not want Jim taking supplements, except for folic acid, Jim felt strongly about taking vitamin C and digestive enzyme-acidophilus. He didn't know any integrative physicians who could help advise him on the safety of supplements, so beyond that, he focused primarily on getting his extra nutrients from food.

**Waiting for Results**
From the very beginning, Jim made the decision that his illness was not going to take him out. There was no way he was going to let himself succumb to the cancer. And even though the doctors told him he would have it for life, and treated it like a chronic disease, Jim was determined to prove his doctors wrong. After a certain number of treatments, his doctors performed scans that showed Jim was doing well and responding to the treatment. Three weeks after his first round of treatment, the size of his tumor had been reduced by 30 percent.

When the tumor shrank so much they found no evidence of it on his spleen and his lymph nodes were back to normal, his doctors declared that the cancer in his bone marrow was low-grade. However, they declared that it was not going to go away. They said they would watch Jim's tests and treat him as needed.

Since chemotherapy was going so well, his doctors backed off his treatment and performed a bone marrow biopsy to determine how many cancer cells remained.

While Jim and Suzanne waited for the results, they decided to get away and have some fun with friends in Colorado. The doctor asked Jim to call him in a couple of days when the results would be in. But they didn't want to hear the bad news that they were expecting and decided to call after their trip was over. Then when they got home they didn't call for a couple of weeks because they were busy, and Jim was back to work.

When Suzanne eventually called, she learned that the bone marrow test came back clean.

Jim was cancer-free. Within a year!

However, although Jim was in remission, he wasn't free to go. The doctor made sure that Jim and Suzanne understood that this type of cancer would surely come back, and Jim was ordered to come in for regular scans. On the one hand, Jim and Suzanne were elated to learn that Jim was cancer free. On the other hand, the doctor's ominous tone about Jim's future prognosis was frightening.

Jim had to be checked every three months — a process that included blood work, a scan, and an exam. After the first year and half, he was allowed to come back once every six months. Then once a year. Finally, by his tenth year, Jim's doctor said that he would prefer to stop doing the scans, as they were now more of a danger in causing cancer than in determining whether it had come back.

Jim was released with the instruction that if he noticed any bumps anywhere he would immediately come back. After ten years of having to be closely watched by his doctors, he was set free.

**Getting It Right**

Jim has remained cancer-free for 16 years. He has also healed emotionally. When Jim got sick he rediscovered his relationship with God and read the Bible cover-to-cover. He focused on his relationships with people. He improved his attitude. He also realized that one of the most important things he could do to heal emotionally was to forgive his mother.

At long last, he was able to let go of the anger and resentment that he had been hanging onto for years and, he was convinced, was making him sick. He became more focused on his faith, family and forgiveness.

Now, Jim's life is divided. There's before cancer and after cancer. While eating healthy food and exercising is important for healing, if he's stressed out and his heart is broken, it's not enough. Jim has been able to heal emotionally and spiritually and find a peaceful balance in life.

**A Gift from God**

Seven years after Jim completed his treatment, after 20 years of marriage to Suzanne, they learned that she was pregnant. Their son, Matthew, was born healthy and happy and is now seven.

Suzanne and Jim have told Matthew about Jim's battle with cancer.

And they have told him that the name Matthew means gift from God.

Suzanne had a recent conversation with Jim's oncologist. She told him, "You said Jim would never go into remission and he did. You said the cancer would never leave his bone marrow and it did. You said we would never have kids, and we have!" The doctor admitted he was wrong. And he expressed how thrilled he was to be proven wrong in this way.

Jim is now 53. He feels better than ever. He has plenty of energy and is in great shape, both physically and emotionally. From his appearance, you would be hard pressed to believe that this strong, masculine, healthy man had gone through such a debilitating disease.

Jim says that getting cancer was the best gift he ever received, because it forced him to straighten out his life. It allowed him to develop a closer relationship with God and the people he loves. At the same time, he always adds that it's a gift — one that he wants to never receive again. He got the lesson and heard the message loud and clear.

*"I help cancer survivors move past their fear of cancer returning and live with joy and confidence by reclaiming their health."*
— *Suzanne (www.vibrantlifeaftercancer.com)*

# *Lymphoma (Non-Hodgkin's Lymphoma) Facts*

*"There is much evidence that cancer is a preventable disease. Only 5–10% of all cancer cases can be attributed to genetic defects, whereas the remaining 90–95% have their roots in the environment and lifestyle."*
*— US National Library of Medicine, National Institutes of Health Pharm Res. Sep 2008; 25(9): 2097–2116*

---

## What Is Lymphoma?

Lymphoma is a type of blood cancer that occurs when lymphocytes (white blood cells that help protect the body from infection and disease) begin behaving abnormally. Abnormal lymphocytes may divide faster than normal cells, may live longer than they are supposed to and may develop in many parts of the body, including the lymph nodes, spleen, bone marrow, blood, or other organs. There are two main types of lymphomas:

1. Hodgkin's lymphoma (HL) that involves the Reed-Sternberg cells
2. Non-Hodgkin's lymphoma (NHL) that does not involve Reed-Sternberg cells.

Non-Hodgkin's lymphoma is divided into four stages, based on how far the disease has spread.

- Stage I (early disease): The cancer is found only in a single lymph node or in one organ or area outside the lymph node.
- Stage II (locally advanced disease): The cancer is found in two or more lymph node regions on one side of the diaphragm.
- Stage III (advanced disease): The cancer involves lymph nodes both above and below the diaphragm.
- Stage IV (widespread disease): The cancer is found in several parts of one or more organs or tissues (in addition to the lymph nodes). Or, it is in the liver, blood, or bone marrow.

## Warning Signs and Symptoms

Certain symptoms are not specific to lymphoma and are similar to those of many other illnesses, including respiratory infections. Common symptoms include:

- Swelling of lymph nodes, which may or may not be painless.
- Fever.
- Unexplained weight loss.

- Sweating (often at night).
- Chills.
- Lack of energy.
- Itching.

While most people who have these symptoms will not have lymphoma, it is important that anyone with persistent symptoms be examined by a doctor.

**Statistics**
Non-Hodgkin's lymphoma (NHL) is one of the most common cancers in the United States, accounting for about 4 percent of all cancers. The American Cancer Society's most recent estimates for NHL for 2014 are:
- About 70,800 people (38,270 males and 32,530 females) will be diagnosed with NHL. This includes both adults and children.
- About 18,990 people will die from this cancer (10,470 males and 8,520 females).

The average American's risk of developing NHL during his or her lifetime is about 1 in 50. Number of new cases and deaths per 100,000: The number of new cases of NHL was 19.7 per 100,000 men and women per year. The number of deaths was 6.3 per 100,000 men and women per year. These rates are age-adjusted and based on 2007–2011 cases and deaths.

Lifetime risk of developing cancer: Approximately 2.1 percent of men and women will be diagnosed with NHL at some point during their lifetime, based on 2009–2011 data. Prevalence of this cancer: In 2011, there were an estimated 530,919 people living with NHL in the United States.

**Further Resources and Helpful Websites**
Lymphoma Research Foundation (www.lymphoma.org)
National Cancer Institute at the National Institute of Health (www.cancer.gov)
American Cancer Society (www.cancer.org)

## 13
# *Rachael Emerges a Victor,*
# *Instead of a Victim*

*"I would never wish the cancer on anybody, but I would never take it back. I wouldn't be where I am today without all of the things that I have been through. It changes you, it makes you more compassionate, it forces you to think twice before doing anything, it pushes you to embrace more in your life."*
*— Rachael Coburn*

### Beautiful, Healthy, and Happy

Rachael is a gorgeous, full of life, and radiant woman who turns heads when she walks down the street. Her husband, Ron, first noticed her just after she finished high school. It was at a New Year's party where he approached Rachael as soon as she walked through the door. They've been together ever since.

Falling in love with Rachael was easy and felt natural. They were young, beautiful, healthy, happily in love, and had no idea what life had in store for them.

### Exhausted, Unwell, and Confused

Rachael left home at 18 for college. She wanted to study medicine, so she became a premed student. In her first year, Rachael started getting sick for no apparent reason. She seemed to catch anything and everything. Moreover, it took weeks to recover from minor illnesses, rather than the few days or a week that she'd been used to. To make things more complicated, simple colds would turn into sinus infections, then into ear infections. Her doctors chalked it up to a new environment and being exposed to new germs. They kept prescribing antibiotics.

Rachael was also tired all the time. Her doctors said it was likely due to the hard work that goes along with being in college, adding that being tired was normal.

Next came the itching. It was constant, mostly where Rachael's bones were close to her skin: her sternum, her lower legs, her scalp. She scratched hard, sometimes in her sleep. Occasionally she would scratch through several layers of her skin. Covered in scabs, she found it difficult to focus on her schoolwork. When she went to see her doctors for help, they suggested changing her soap and lotion. And they prescribed steroids to address the itching.

Initially, the steroids helped. However, when she was done taking them, within a week or two the itching would start up again. At this point, no one felt there was anything significant going on. Then Rachael started to have night sweats. Despite the cold temperature in her room, she would wake up so sweaty that she'd need to change her clothes. She blamed the nightmares she was having. And lastly, she would get very sick and dizzy from drinking the smallest amount of alcohol. Even one sip made her vomit.

All this went on for 18 months.

**Putting the Pieces Together**
As a first-year premed student, Rachael's symptoms hadn't come up in her curriculum yet. In her second year, she began to realize that she was suffering from something significant.

Then, in the shower, she felt something in her armpit. It felt like a golf ball. Rachael immediately thought back through every moment that she didn't feel well. She realized that this was why she was constantly pulling out her shirtsleeves, stretching the armpit. Why she was always adjusting her blouses for feeling too tight under her arm. Everything came sharply into focus — the night sweats, the rash, the constant colds and infections, the tiredness. She had cancer.

She went straight from the shower to her computer. The first thing that came up was lymphoma. She realized that she had it in her armpits and neck. She knew that everything in her neck was swollen. The back of her skull had masses. Under her chin and clavicle.

She was shocked that this went on for so long. How could she not notice this, she wondered. With her one discovery in the shower, it took less than five minutes to put it all together.

**Conventional Care as the Cornerstone of Treatment**
Rachael's doctors performed a CT scan and sent her to a hospital in Boston a few times to confirm the diagnosis, learn the stage of her cancer, and determine her treatment.

She had Hodgkin's lymphoma, they told her. It hadn't crossed her diaphragm, but they did see some lesions on her liver. Her condition was classified as stage 2B, which means full-blown symptoms: fever, rashes, weight loss, and night sweats. She would receive chemotherapy in Boston: six rounds of ABVD, a regimen commonly used in the first-line treatment of Hodgkin's lymphoma.

However, immediately after her first transfusion, she experienced an adverse reaction to Bleomycin, the B part of ABVD. She developed lung and heart damage as a result, and this part of the treatment was taken out right away. Her oncologists extended the duration of her chemotherapy regiment to account for the adjustment.

Rachael struggled with chemotherapy, which she received every two weeks. She felt very sick after each round, with continuing nausea. Each time she had to go back, she was terrified, knowing how bad she would feel afterward.

Partway in, Rachael developed a severe rash all over her body, which she self-diagnosed as shingles. Her doctor didn't believe her, saying that people can only get shingles in one quadrant of their body — and Rachael had it from head to toe. At Rachael's insistence, the doctor tested her. The lab results came back indicating that she did indeed have shingles. And it meant she would need to skip chemotherapy for that month.

After her treatment was over, Rachael continued to get CT scans every three months. Within the following year, her oncologist told her that the cancer had come back to her small intestine. He suggested that she "get her affairs in order." She was not yet 21 years old, and thought to herself: "what affairs do I have?"

The doctors were considering giving Rachael salvage chemotherapy, which is a rescue therapy, a form of treatment given after an ailment does not respond to standard treatment. Rachael, in the meantime, began looking at the possibility of receiving a bone marrow transplant from her twin sister. The doctors were considering all the options, but Rachael didn't feel like they were helping. She didn't get the support and encouragement she expected from her doctors. And that was when Rachael went home and decided that she had to take action.

### Becoming Her Own Superhero and Taking Her Health into Her Own Hands

She had to do something about her condition, but what? First, Rachael saw an acupuncturist, which she hoped would make her feel stronger. Next, she read Beating Cancer with Nutrition by Patrick Quillin. Rachael was so taken with the book — and quite frankly so desperate for options — that she followed it religiously. She started to eat "cleanly" because of the connection between cancer and sugar. Immediately, she eliminated all the sugar in her house.

From that point on, nothing went into her mouth that wasn't "food as a medicine." Every bite had to have some healing properties, nutritional values, anticancer properties, antioxidants, or anti-inflammatory powers. She felt that, if nothing else, it would make her stronger in the event that she would need another round of chemotherapy.

When her oncologist scheduled more treatment a few weeks out, Rachael asked for a biopsy to make sure that the treatment was really needed. Her doctors complied, and also scheduled an endoscopy to check her small intestine.

That endoscopy was done just a month after Rachael started her new, rigid eating routine. It was one month of eating cancer-killing foods and taking extra-special care of herself — one month of determination to become well.

After the test, her doctors were stunned. They couldn't find the tumor. They weren't sure whether something went wrong with the machine. And Rachael didn't care how the "conventional medical" world would explain what had just happened. She went home and kept doing what she was doing.

In a month, when she went back to do another PET/CT scan, they once again could not see anything. So once again, Rachael left home and continued eating her way out of the cancer. It gave her a sense of power and control over her own health. And it made her feel stronger — not only physically, but also emotionally.

Rachael continued to be monitored every month. Eventually, the time between her checkups was extended to every three months. Then to every six months. And after three years, Rachael didn't have to come back for a check-up for a full year. Today, 15 years later, her scans are over, and she continues to get blood work done annually.

## Life After Cancer

After being declared cancer free, Rachael continued to follow her strict diet for a few years. She made juices with greens. She didn't eat meat. And she ate no sugar, except for fruit sugar in small amounts. But no processed sugar, not even honey or maple syrup. She didn't want to feed the cancer in case there were any cancer cells left. Then eventually, she started eating a less strict diet, while keeping it clean and organic.

She continued to fear that her cancer might come back. After every check-up, her doctors would increase the interval between visits. That freedom made her feel afraid. She wondered, what if something happened in those months? She had to rely on her belief that she'd be able to rescue herself if there was a need.

## Starting a Family

When Rachael became well and strong enough, she and her boyfriend, Ron, decided to get married. They hadn't considered having a family because the chemotherapy had put Rachael into suspected menopause. They kind of let go of the idea of ever having children. They were just happy that Rachael was alive and they were together.

When they returned from their honeymoon, Rachael was surprised to discover that she was pregnant. It was wonderful news for them. And scary. However, very early on, Rachael lost that pregnancy. Her doctor told her that lots of women lose their first pregnancy, and it was nothing to be concerned about. She assured Rachael and Ron not to think twice about it.

A few months later, Rachael got pregnant again. Eight weeks in, at a checkup, her doctors found no heartbeat. It was Rachael's second miscarriage, but her doctor still told her not to worry. She should only be worried after miscarrying for the third time. Very shortly after that, she miscarried again.

Now, Rachael decided to look into the matter and determine why this was happening. She was examined and told that there was nothing wrong with her fallopian tubes. Her uterus and ovaries were fine. The doctors admitted that they didn't know why she was miscarrying.

She was given a green light to try again and got pregnant for the fourth time. This time, the baby was stillborn at 22 weeks. An examination revealed that the baby had full triploidy, an extremely rare chromosomal disorder where a fetus has three copies of every chromosome.

Rachael felt that the mutation was most likely from her being exposed to so much radiation when she was going through cancer treatment. Even after she was cancer free, she was still getting regular scans and had a lot of exposure to radiation. The doctors agreed that was probably the root of the problem. While they hoped it wouldn't happen again, there was no guarantee.

When Rachael got pregnant for the fifth time, everything seemed to be going well. This time around Rachael was particularly cautious and saw her doctor every two weeks to be checked. Soon she felt that something was wrong and told to her doctor about her fears. The doctor wouldn't take her concerns seriously.

Sure enough, when Rachael went for her twelve-week appointment, the baby's heart had stopped. All the doctor could say was to admit that Rachael was right and there was something wrong.

Rachael's sixth pregnancy turned out to be another very early loss.

At this point Rachael and Ron were so defeated they thought they weren't meant to have children. Then they considered in vitro fertilization (IVF), which is the process of fertilization by manually combining an egg and sperm in a laboratory dish, and then transferring the embryo to the uterus. That would allow them to have preimplantation genetic diagnosis, a reproductive technology used to diagnose genetic diseases in early embryos prior to implantation and pregnancy. They would rather find out right away whether the child would be viable than to carry it and find out later.

They started IVF preparation and genetic testing. Through this, they found out that Rachael had mutations in her methylation cycle, specifically with regard to folate metabolism. So these mutations didn't allow her to properly utilize B vitamins, particularly folic acid.

The doctor said that Rachael would be able to carry a baby to term if she prepared her body and supported her pregnancy with activated B vitamins, aspirin, and natural progesterone, along with eating organic and nutritionally dense foods.

Then, before they began the actual IVF, Rachael got pregnant again. This was the seventh time. Luckily, they had already discussed the protocol of using the activated B vitamins, progesterone, and aspirin. So she started to use them right away through her pregnancy.

When Rachael was at 21 weeks, she started to feel contractions. She was rushed to the hospital and told that she had irritable uterus, where her body was considering expelling the baby due to irritation. Rachael was contracting all the time. She followed up with her regular doctor to ask for help stopping the contractions, as she was concerned that she'd go into labor. The doctor said that there was not lot of available research on that subject.

She got a second opinion and was told they may want to simply remove the fetus, because it's likely that there was an infection in there. That infection might have been the reason for irritation, and there was no way to tell without doing amniocentesis or removing the fetus. Rachael still shakes her head when she recalls this conversation, calling it the most ridiculous thing she had ever heard.

This was one of the many times when Rachael felt that the doctors were looking at her like she was a box on a factory shelf. Rachael was determined to have this baby, no matter what! So she put herself on bed rest and pulled herself together with the same energy that she used to battle cancer. From that moment on, everything she put into her mouth was to heal her baby. She ate garlic, asparagus, and poached eggs. She drank green tea, took supplements, consumed probiotics, vitamin D, and everything she could possibly find online that would calm an infection from an irritable uterus. Everything that would support a healthy pregnancy. Everything that would support strong membranes.

She was on bed rest for the three months. She had help from her family and was only able to get up to go to bathroom. Everybody made her meals and took care of her and of the house.

At 36 weeks, she started to have the contractions again. However, once she got through 36 weeks, she knew that the baby was strong enough to come out and would survive. So Rachael started getting up and moving around.

Ironically this baby ended up not getting out on time. Madeline was finally born at 41 weeks. It was a beautiful, natural delivery. Two years later, while she was still nursing Madeline, Rachael got pregnant again.

She and Ron wanted to have another child, but thought that it might be another uneasy pregnancy, so they had hoped to wait until their daughter Madeline got a bit older. However, they embraced the news and were ready to do all they could to make it through.

Thankfully, this was a beautiful pregnancy. Rachael knew what she had to do and right away started taking activated B vitamins, the natural progesterone, and aspirin. She ate a supportive and restrictive diet with no dairy and no gluten — all organic. Rachael believes this contributed to how easy this pregnancy went. It was so simple, she could forget that she was pregnant.

While this pregnancy was super easy, the delivery was tough. The baby stopped moving, and the doctors couldn't find her heartbeat for a moment, so they conducted an emergency C-section. While Rachael was hoping for a natural delivery, she was thankful because that was the time where a surgeon was needed. And Emma was born.

### Empowered, Healthy and Happy
It's been 15 years since Rachael was diagnosed with cancer and 14 since she's been cancer free. Today she enjoys the confidence that comes with knowing she can take care of herself and her family. While she has the support of integrative and naturopathic doctors, Rachael feels secure with her own knowledge and gained skills.

Her beautiful daughters are five and three. Rachael makes sure that they eat a "clean" diet in and out of their house. The girls take homemade lunches to school. When they eat treats, they're color/chemical/ antibiotics/ steroids/gluten–free sweets that are now widely available in health-food stores.

### Whole Body Integrative Approach Versus a Conventional "Conveyer" Tactic
In Rachael's experience, many doctors simply attempted to suppress her symptoms without paying attention to why the symptoms were there. There would be little investigation into what was happening with the rest of her body. The naturopathic and integrative-health practitioners she saw, on the other hand, looked at her whole body and searched for why, which is the most important piece of the puzzle.

At the point in Rachael's life when she got sick, she wanted to become a doctor. After her ordeal, she realized that doctors aren't the superheroes she'd always thought they were. They're just people who are able to implement what they are taught.

If there is one lesson to take from Rachael's courageous journey, let it be this: there are times when there are no superheroes to rescue you, other than you. Your health is in your hands.

Rachael admits that while she would never wish cancer on others, she wouldn't trade her experience for anything. She wouldn't be where she is today without what she went through. It changed her; it made her more compassionate; it forced her to think twice before doing anything; and it pushed her to embrace more in her life.

---

*"We need to make sure we are changing the medical community so they are taught and trained to understand the very reason why someone is sick. Not just what's wrong with the person, but why is it happening."*
*— Rachael (www.ctwellnessandweightloss.com)*

# Hodgkin's Lymphoma Facts

*"Lymphoma is the most common blood cancer, with more than 65,000 new cases diagnosed each year in the United States alone. It has taken the lives of such people as former First Lady Jackie Kennedy Onassis, baseball great Roger Maris, country western icon Gene Autry, punk rocker Joey Ramone and flying legend Charles Lindbergh. But lymphoma, in its various forms, still does not receive the amount of public attention or financial support that many other cancers receive."*
— *Jamie Reno, author, cancer survivor*

## What Is Lymphoma?

Lymphoma is a type of blood cancer that occurs when lymphocytes (white blood cells that help protect the body from infection and disease) begin behaving abnormally. Abnormal lymphocytes may divide faster than normal cells, may live longer than they are supposed to and may develop in many parts of the body, including the lymph nodes, spleen, bone marrow, blood, or other organs. There are two main types of lymphomas:

- Hodgkin's lymphoma (HL) that involves the Reed-Sternberg cells
- Non-Hodgkin's lymphoma (NHL) that does not involve Reed-Sternberg cells.

Hodgkin's lymphoma begins when a lymphocyte (usually a B cell) becomes abnormal (Reed-Sternberg cell).

## Warning Signs and Symptoms

The first sign of Hodgkin's disease is often an enlarged lymph node. The disease can spread to nearby lymph nodes, to the lungs, liver, or bone marrow. Other Symptoms include:

- Painless swelling of the lymph nodes in the neck, armpits, or groin
- Fever and chills
- Night sweats
- Weight loss
- Loss of appetite
- Itchy skin
- Lack of energy

These symptoms are nonspecific and could be caused by a number of

93

conditions unrelated to cancer. However, in lymphoma, the symptoms persist over time and cannot be explained by an infection or another disease.

**Statistics**
- The number of new cases of Hodgkin's lymphoma was 2.7 per 100,000 men and women per year. The number of deaths was 0.4 per 100,000 men and women per year. These rates are age-adjusted and based on 2007-2011 cases and deaths.
- Approximately 0.2 percent of men and women will be diagnosed with Hodgkin's lymphoma at some point during their lifetime, based on 2009-2011 data.
- In 2011, there were an estimated 185,793 people living with Hodgkin's lymphoma in the United States.

**Further Resources and Helpful Websites**
American Cancer Fund
(americancancerfund.org/cancer-types/lymphoma/ lymphoma – symptoms)
National Institutes of Health
(www.nlm.nih.gov/medlineplus/hodgkindisease.html)
National Cancer Institute (www.cancer.gov/statfacts/html/hodg.html)

## *14*
## *Strong Enough to Live This Life*

*"To everyone who is battling cancer — KEEP FIGHTING.*
*Dig deep and give it everything you've got.*
*You are way stronger than you realize. Every day is a new battle, the hardest*
*battle you'll ever encounter in your life.*
*But no matter what, know that you are going to beat it.*
*Wake up every day knowing that your mission is to come out on top.*
*Even if the light at the end of that tunnel seems far, it's there.*
*Keep your head held high and a smile on your face, even when it hurts.*
*That in itself will make more of a difference than you know.*

*To those of you who know someone fighting the fight — DON'T BE AFRAID.*
*Don't be scared to talk to that person and*
*don't be scared to be there for them.*
*When you're unsure about something, it's easy to think the worst.*
*Sometimes it's even easier to take a step back in fear of losing that person forever.*
*Don't. Chances are, their battle will be harder for you than it is for them.*

*To those of you that have lost someone to cancer — REMEMBER THE GOOD*
*TIMES,*
*even if at times it's hard. Take their strength with you everywhere you go, and use*
*that every day to continue to have fun and be happy.*

*To those who have won the battle — the fighters who*
*gave it their all each and every day, those who never gave up and never took "No" for*
*an answer, you are truly special.*
*Chances are you knew you were going to beat it the entire time ...*
*YOU ARE TRULY AMAZING."*

*— TJ Carbone*

To celebrate his 25th birthday, TJ spent the entire weekend partying with his friends. The following Monday, he woke up and couldn't roll over in bed. He felt something odd on his neckline and saw in the mirror what looked like a ball on his neck. He knew it was his lymph node, but attributed it to partying too much.

At work, his colleagues looked at the mass on TJ's neck with alarm.

Someone said that they knew somebody with the exact same thing, and

95

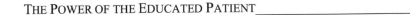

that it was cancer. TJ was definitely not accepting that. However, he was concerned enough to call a doctor right away.

The next day he had an x-ray taken and asked the doctor what could it be, worst-case scenario. She hesitated at first. Then she admitted that she had seen this sort of thing before. Worst-case scenario, she told him, is that it could be lymphoma. This seemed unreal to TJ, and he immediately texted his good friends and his mom.

**Not Knowing, Not Sure, and Not in Control**
In the days that followed, TJ couldn't think straight and couldn't eat. Then, he got a call from the doctor. She said the report came out perfectly fine and there was nothing to worry about. Nevertheless, there was huge mass around TJ's neck and he needed to figure out what it was.

Later that day he went back to the doctor's office and was told that he needed to have a biopsy done. TJ was shocked, as he was previously told that there was nothing major.

It took a few days after the biopsy was performed to get the results.

**Looking the Doctor in the Eyes**
TJ's mom flew down from Connecticut and went with TJ to learn the biopsy results. When the doctor came out, he looked TJ right in the eyes and told him that he had cancer. The cancer was pushing against everything inside his chest and everything from his heart to esophagus was being affected. His official diagnosis was Advanced Bulky Stage 2 Hodgkin's Lymphoma.

TJ had just turned 25 and thought he had experienced every feeling the world had to offer. On this day, he discovered he was wrong. It was one of those moments that you pray never happens to you or anyone you know. One of those days that really makes you put things into perspective and look at life in a completely different way.

TJ's head was spinning. The scariest part was not knowing what was going to happen — not knowing what he was in for. It was the first time as an adult that he wasn't in control. TJ's mom asked the oncologist: if it were his son what would he do? The doctor said that he would put his son on a plane, get him home, and get the process moving.

That evening, TJ's friends came over to his condo and helped him pack.

To give himself time to think, he drove the whole way from Florida to Connecticut.

## Sorry Cancer, Did You Really Think You Stood a Chance?
When TJ learned more about his disease and what was going to happen in treatment, all of his anxiety, nervousness, and stress went away. It really wasn't a big deal anymore as it was clear to him that dying wasn't an option. He knew he was going to beat cancer.

To stay focused, he visualized a day in the future, after his treatment and recovery, his doctor shaking his hand, looking him right in the eye and telling him that he is good — that he beat it.

To make that happen, he just needed to know what to do to get better. He wanted to know everything about cancer. He made it a point to spend as much time as possible reading, researching, asking questions, learning, and experimenting. And he recorded all of it along the way. The one thing he was missing was a "Here's what you're about to go through, what to do, how to deal with it" how-to guide.

## Therapy
At his first appointment at Yale–New Haven Hospital, he received a PET scan and everything he needed to start chemotherapy the next week. Another bump had formed on the other side of his neck, so he also had another biopsy performed.

After having done as much research as possible, he knew he was going to start chemo right away. He knew what kind of chemo he was going to do before his doctor even told him.

TJ went through the whole chemotherapy process. Once every two weeks for five months — 12 sessions total. Going through chemo was terrible, but he scheduled dates and events with others to keep his spirits up. He believes it was way harder for his family and friends. In about two months and after only four treatments of chemo, TJ was in remission. No cancer.

At what would be his very last treatment, six months in, he felt that his body had had enough. He followed his heart and instinct and opted out of that last treatment. He also decided against doing radiation. He read a great deal about radiation and decided that he didn't want any more drugs or anything bad going into his body.

When TJ told his oncologist — one of the best specialists at Yale who has been practicing for a very long time — that he didn't want to do last round, the doctor recommended against that, telling him it's what he's supposed to do and all the clinical studies are based on huge groups of people doing the same things. He also suggested that TJ meet with the radiation oncologist before making his decision about radiation.

Although TJ was 100 percent confident on not doing radiation, he met the radiologist and asked to see exactly where the radiation would be going. It was around his heart. TJ bristled, because he knew about the secondary type of cancer that could come after doing radiation.

TJ felt that, for doctors, cancer is a numbers game that needs to be played by the book. To get individual attention across the board one really has to go out of his way and meet with tons of other doctors and people that have gone through it and learn along the way.

When TJ had a follow-up PET scan, he was told that he was still in remission and everything was okay. The picture of his oncologist shaking his hand, looking him in the eyes and saying that he is cancer free came to reality. Exactly the way TJ envisioned it!

**Back to a New Normal**
Today, feeling "normal" is wonderful for TJ. It's a new feeling, and he's definitely not at the place he was before his diagnosis. While he is back to his busy life and friends, he makes sure he is taking way better care of himself.

What makes TJ feel better is regular exercise, yoga, meditation, breathing techniques, acupuncture, and detox baths. More important than those, however, are his changed lifestyle and diet. He learned that the better he eats, the better he feels. What used to be burger and fries for breakfast is now sweet potato, kale, onion, and garlic. He used to complain that waking up in the morning and getting out of the bed was hard. Today, he totally appreciates waking up in the morning and not having to follow a schedule for getting his blood work done or going in for chemo appointments. Instead, he's able to do what he wants, when he wants.

TJ used to go to sleep at three or four in the morning. Today he makes sure he goes to sleep at a reasonable time, and when he gets up in the morning he jumps out of bed rested and ready for the day — something he never felt before.

TJ also appreciates his relationships even more. He pays more attention to his day-to-day surroundings. He's become fearless in new situations. He's quick to introduce himself to strangers, has no qualms about moving to a new city and starting a new job, and has chosen to travel out of the country for a new experience.

For TJ, what it all comes down to is a positive attitude. Staying upbeat, doing whatever's necessary to overcome obstacles, keeping a smile on his face — even on days when it hurts to open his eyes — are what it's all about. He believes that if you create positive thoughts, they become your reality. When you start really thinking positively, things start to change for the better. The thoughts we have and the stories we tell ourselves become the way we live our lives.

Overcoming cancer wasn't just a battle TJ won, it was an experience he'll always remember and live by. Every moment is a chance to learn, to try, and to do new things. Everything he learned over the course of the last six months is helping him blaze a new trail forward.

---

*"So now it's your turn. Take your first step toward whatever it is that you want right now. 'F' all the noise — no one is going to do it for you. Deep down, you've gotta really want it, and know you'll get it. And always ... believe in you."*

*— TJ (www.facebook.com/tjcarbon)*

# Hodgkin's Lymphoma Facts

*"Many people enjoy long and healthy lives after being successfully treated for Hodgkin's lymphoma. Sometimes, however, the treatment can affect a person's health for months or even years after it has finished. The long-termor late effects and can include fertility problems, a higher risk of developing a secondary cancer later in life, as well as cardiac and gut problems."*
— *Leukemia Foundation*

## What Is Lymphoma?

Lymphoma is a type of blood cancer that occurs when lymphocytes (white blood cells that help protect the body from infection and disease) begin behaving abnormally. Abnormal lymphocytes may divide faster than normal cells, may live longer than they are supposed to and may develop in many parts of the body, including the lymph nodes, spleen, bone marrow, blood, or other organs. There are two main types of lymphomas:

1. Hodgkin's lymphoma (HL) that involves the Reed-Sternberg cells
2. Non-Hodgkin's lymphoma (NHL) that does not involve Reed-Sternberg cells.

Hodgkin's lymphoma begins when a lymphocyte (usually a B cell) becomes abnormal (Reed-Sternberg cell).

## Warning Signs and Symptoms

The first sign of Hodgkin's disease is often an enlarged lymph node. The disease can spread to nearby lymph nodes, to the lungs, liver, or bone marrow. Other Symptoms include:

- Painless swelling of the lymph nodes in the neck, armpits, or groin
- Fever and chills
- Night sweats
- Weight loss
- Loss of appetite
- Itchy skin
- Lack of energy

These symptoms are nonspecific and could be caused by a number of conditions unrelated to cancer. However, in lymphoma, the symptoms persist over time and cannot be explained by an infection or another disease.

**Statistics**

The number of new cases of Hodgkin's lymphoma was 2.7 per 100,000 men and women per year. The number of deaths was 0.4 per 100,000 men and women per year. These rates are age-adjusted and based on 2007-2011 cases and deaths.

Approximately 0.2 percent of men and women will be diagnosed with Hodgkin's lymphoma at some point during their lifetime, based on 2009-2011 data.

In 2011, there were an estimated 185,793 people living with Hodgkin's lymphoma in the United States.

**Further Resources and Helpful Websites**

AmericanCancerFund
(www.americancancerfund.org/cancer-types/lymphoma/lymphoma-symptoms)
National Institutes of Health
(www.nlm.nih.gov/medlineplus/ hodgkindisease.html)
National Cancer Institute
(www.cancer.gov/statfacts/html/hodg.html)

*Part V*

*Primary Immunodeficiency Disorders*

## 15
## *From Chronically Ill to Healthy and Vibrant*

*By Dr. Karen Moriarty*

*"You need to be proactive, carve out time in your schedule, and take responsibility for being the healthiest person you can be - no one else is going to do it for you."*
*— Dr Mehmet Oz*

### The Beginning of the Learning Journey
Karen's journey toward her vocation as a chiropractor began when she was one of those kids who was always sick. She was prescribed so many rounds of penicillin for strep throat that her doctors finally removed her tonsils at the tender age of six. They expected that it would make her healthier. But it did no such thing — her body just found other ways to be sick.

By age 12, Karen was 20 pounds underweight, had difficulty sleeping, and suffered from chronic digestive issues and debilitating menstrual cramps. She suffered multiple colds, flus, and bouts of sore throat every winter. Prescriptions were filled and taken like clockwork. She thought this was normal.

Out of desperation, Karen's doctors removed her appendix, even though she did not have appendicitis. Her ailing physical state began to take a toll on her emotions. She became chronically anxious. She bit her nails down to the quick. Her hands shook like those of an advanced Parkinson's patient.

In every way possible, Karen's health progressively declined throughout her childhood. She didn't know it, but she'd become a poster child for what's wrong with our medical care system; that trying to heal through pharmaceuticals doesn't work; that a healthy body can only be created by a healthy lifestyle.

The turning point for Karen came in her junior year of high school. She took a job as a nurse's aide in a nursing home and fell in love with taking care of people. While she continued this type of employment through college, she became increasingly troubled by what she witnessed: overly medicated patients, the insanity of feeding sick people processed non-nutritious foods, and doctors spending very little time caring for and interacting with their patients. Because of this, she chose to steer clear of pursuing a career as a nurse or medical doctor.

Instead, she pursued a pre-medical degree in biology. And the more she learned, the more she began to care for her own body — in more natural ways. When Karen became sick, she now took supplements because she found that she recovered quicker and didn't experience any of the unpleasant negative effects of medications. She looked at her overall diet and ate more whole foods. She even read a few good nutrition books — now considered old school — by Adelle Davis and Dr. Feingold.

Karen also began to realize that her spirit and personality were probably not well suited for a career where she'd be confined to a science lab. But she didn't know what else she could do that would allow her to participate in the world that she knew she belonged in: health care.

**Something Different**
Then, during her last semester of pre-med, a close friend injured his spine at work, developed agonizing back pain, and begged her to take him to a chiropractor. Karen tried to talk him into going to a local medical center instead, but he refused. He told her that he had previously suffered from severe lower-back pain, and after six weeks of taking prescribed drugs and getting recommended bed rest, he saw no improvement. So he went to a chiropractor, and he recovered rapidly. Completely skeptical, Karen took him to a chiropractic office near her school.

When they arrived, Karen helped him into the reception area and looked around. Between the warm welcome from the staff, the thoughtful decor, and the informational posters, something felt different. She felt the kindness and concern of the doctors and staff, and she knew that this was a defining moment in her life.

When Karen's friend's first visit was over, he felt significant relief, delivered by safe and effective hands-on care. Karen was fascinated. After a few more visits, Karen had the privilege of speaking with other patients, the staff, and then finally the doctor. She looks back now and realizes that chiropractic had her at "hello."

**A New Path**
Karen discovered the world of vitalism, or the understanding that in all living creatures there's an innate intelligence with a far greater capacity for healing and vitality than science will ever attain, and she immediately felt at home.

Suddenly, everything that Karen had observed while working in nursing homes and hospitals and learned in her pre-med studies made more sense. She knew in her core that there were aspects of health, healing, and vitality that could not be explained by random biochemical reactions and DNA. Karen had witnessed patients fully recover from serious diseases through lifestyle changes — but never through medications and surgery alone.

Thankfully, she followed this new path and went to Chiropractic College. And as she received frequent chiropractic care and learned more about nutrition, exercise, and stress reduction, she became healthier than she had ever been. Her journey continues to this day.

---

*"Our purpose is to educate and adjust as many families as possible to optimal health through natural chiropractic care."*

*— Dr.Karen (www.northborochiropractic.com)*

# *Immunodeficiency (Immune Deficiency) Facts*

*"Primary immunodeficiency disorders —weaken the immune system, allowing infections and other health problems to occur more easily."*
*— Mayo Clinic*

## What Is Immunodeficiency (or "chronically ill")
Immunodeficiency (or immune deficiency) is a state in which the immune system's ability to fight infectious disease is compromised or entirely absent.

## Warning Signs and Symptoms (of primary immunodeficiency)
An increased susceptibility to infections that are more frequent, longer lasting or harder to treat than are the infections of someone with a normal immune system.
- Frequent and recurrent pneumonia, bronchitis, sinus infections, ear infections, meningitis or skin infections
- Blood infections
- Inflammation and infection of internal organs
- Blood disorders, such as low platelet counts or anemia
- Digestive problems, such as cramping, loss of appetite, nausea and diarrhea
- Delayed growth and development
- Autoimmune disorders, such as lupus, rheumatoid arthritis or type 1 diabetes

## Karen's Symptoms
- Constant strep throat
- Underweight
- Difficulty sleeping
- Chronic digestive issues
- Debilitating menstrual cramps
- Multiple colds, flus, and throat irritation every winter
- Chronic anxiety

## Statistics
Common variable immunodeficiency (CVID), the most commonly diagnosed primary immunodeficiency, is estimated to affect one in 25,000 to one in 50,000 people worldwide.

## Further Resources and Helpful Websites
http://www.nlm.nih.gov/medlineplus/healthtopics.html

# *Part VI*

# *Chronic Disorders*

## 16
## *When a Book Is Your Magic Wand*

*"Books are a uniquely portable magic."*
— Stephen King

*"Be careful about reading health books. You may die of a misprint."*
— Mark Twain

---

### Unwell and Struggling

An unfortunate car accident caused the retinas in both of Laura's eyes to detach. Emergency surgery repaired the damage, but soon she began experiencing ocular migraines, which caused vision loss for up to an hour, often following a debilitating headache. Then came the visual disturbances weird spiky shapes in front of her face. These episodes were usually triggered by watching TV and could go on for twenty minutes, and then the shapes would just vanish.

Laura's ophthalmologist told her that she had a cataract, a clouding of the lens in her eye. He added that it was an unusual type of cataract for someone in her late 40s. Laura had cataract surgery and her ocular migraine stopped. A few years later, she woke up to a painful, pounding migraine that went on for hours. She got through it, but the following week she had five more. Each time, she could barely move.

These continued to get worse until finally her husband insisted she go to the hospital. By this time Laura's blood pressure was sky high and doctors thought she could be having a heart attack. After testing her heart and scanning her brain, they couldn't find anything wrong. At a loss, they simply gave her a shot of morphine to help with the pain and sent her home. Her husband practically had to carry her from the car into the house.

Laura woke up the next morning and her blood pressure was very high again. Throughout the day, it went down and up. A few days later, she went to see an internist who was also a cardiologist. The doctor said that Laura's migraine was definitely driven by high blood pressure. She put Laura on the lowest dose of a blood pressure medication, suggesting that she take it when she feels a migraine is coming on. This blood pressure medication made Laura feel overwhelmingly dizzy, she couldn't even walk across the room without her knees starting to buckle. And her heart would race each time she took it.

With nowhere else to go, Laura decided to see a Chinese acupuncturist. After an examination, he suggested that she stop taking her blood pressure medication under the guidance of her primary care doctor. He performed acupuncture on her and gave her a combination of Chinese herbs to help with her headaches and anxiety. Within a couple of months, Laura felt good enough that she didn't need to stay on the Chinese herbs any longer.

## Stress

Laura was fine for about 10 years after that. But then she found herself in a very stressful work situation. She began having pain in her lower back, and the back of her legs would get knotted up. At the time, she was seeing a chiropractor who had been adjusting just her upper cervical spine. What he didn't realize was that Laura had a misalignment in her lower, lumbar vertebrae, and the way he was adjusting her was actually making matters worse. Her lumbar spine was not going to fall in line and that's what he was expecting. He was actually pulling the rest of her spine further away from the lumbar vertebrae. Her lower back pain got worse and worse. Then she began to experience dizziness. And she couldn't walk more than 10 to 15 minutes before her feet got numb.

Eventually she left the job and expected her health to improve on its own — but it didn't. So she found a different chiropractic office with a totally different approach. They helped a bit, but the pain still came and went.

## Posture and Stretch Trainings

Soon Laura found a posture expert, Eric Goodman, who does foundation training. Some of the posture-correction movements helped with Laura's low back pain. Apparently her glutes had been spasming for months or even years. And one stretch that she learned set that muscle out, making her feel a lot better. She also took a training developed by another posture expert named Esther Gochale. That allowed her to get even better. However, the vertigo would still come and go.

## The Magic of the Right Book

Laura was determined to find the right cure, and finally someone suggested reading the book *Heal Your Headache* by David Buchholz. The book is based on the theory that virtually all headaches are forms of migraine. Migraine is not a specific type of headache, but the built-in mechanism that causes headaches of all kinds. Buchholz offers a simple solution that includes three main steps:

1. Avoid the *quick fix* of painkillers, as they only make matters worse
2. Reduce the migraine triggers through a diet that eliminates the foods that push headaches
3. Raise the *threshold* with preventive medication

Everyone has their own threshold, and there are people who are more sensitive to the triggers that include certain foods, drugs, and stress. If the triggers stay below that threshold, the person won't get a headache. But if they go over, the person gets a classic migraine headache.

The book suggested the elimination diet, which is used to identify foods that may be causing an adverse effect. So the person excludes all suspected foods from the diet and then reintroduces one at a time. Laura decided to experiment and see if she felt differently by implementing the below elimination diet:

**Migraine Trigger Foods to AVOID\***

- Caffeine Chocolate
- MSG (monosodium glutamate) Processed meats and fish
- Some dairy
  - o aged cheese, sour cream, butter milk, yogurt Nuts and peanuts
- Alcohol and most vinegar, except white distilled Bottled sauces and salad dressings
- Some fruits
  - o raisins, dates, dried fruit with sulfites
  - o citrus (oranges, lemons, limes, grapefruit) and pineapple
  - o bananas, red plums
  - o raspberries, figs
  - o avocado, papayas, passion fruit
- Some vegetables
  - o onions
  - o snow peas, sugar snap peas
  - o some beans: fava beans, lentils, lima beans, navy beans, and broad Italian beans
  - o might want to avoid soy; some soy products may be fine (soybean oil)
  - o some people have problems with tomatoes
  - o some people have problems with peas and mushrooms (high amounts of naturally free glutamate)
  - o

- Fresh yeast-risen products Artificial sweeteners
- Anything else you know is a trigger

After going off most of the migraine triggers, Laura felt better almost immediately. It was close to a miracle. She wondered: Could it really be all due to the food triggers she avoided? To know for sure, one night she ate half a peanut butter sandwich — one of her usual triggers — before bed. She woke up the next morning with a migraine. This was a real turning point for her. After only two months of avoiding her food triggers, Laura felt 90 percent better. Her headache, vertigo, and even back pain were all dramatically reduced.

**Depression and an Active Form of B-12**
What still hadn't been helped was Laura's depression. But she happened to read a thought-provoking book called *Could It Be B12?: An Epidemic of Misdiagnoses* by Sally M. Pacholok and Jeffrey J. Stuart. The book presents a wide scope of problems caused by B12 deficiency and provides up-to-date medical information about symptoms, testing, diagnosis, and treatment.

Laura learned that a B-12 deficiency could have caused almost all of her symptoms. From earlier testing, she was aware that she had deficiencies of B-12 and magnesium, and she was already taking a B-12 supplement. But she discovered that the B-12 supplement she had been taking wasn't the active form of B-12. What she needed was methylcobalmin.

Laura also learned about the importance of magnesium as a treatment for migraines. After she began taking the correct type and dose of magnesium, she felt her whole system calming down. Just a few days after she started taking the combination of active B12 and magnesium, she started to feel better.

The next book that brought Laura closer to recovery was *Younger Next Year: Live Strong, Fit, and Sexy — Until You're 80 and Beyond* by Chris Crowley and Henry S. Lodge. It shows how to turn back our biological clock and delay 70 percent of the normal problems of aging (weakness, sore joints, bad balance) and eliminate 50 percent of serious illness and injury. Following its guidance, Laura began exercising an hour a day, six days a week. The numbness in her feet went away.

Today Laura feels like herself again; she is hopeful and somewhat relieved. If she sits for extended periods of time, she'll still get back pain.

She stopped getting migraines, but can still feel them creeping in sometimes. Over a recent Christmas holiday, she wandered a little too far off her elimination diet. The next day it was obvious that diet still mattered, as she experienced brain fog, migraine tension, vertigo, and ringing in her ears — all from a few indulgent meals.

Laura's back is still misaligned, and that's not going to go away any time soon. But when her migraine symptoms decrease, she doesn't get the spasms that make that misalignment painful. So her muscle pain and inability to walk were the side effects of her migraines.

Laura is a strong believer and an advocate of taking your health in your hands and staying in charge!

---

*"Stay in charge of your health, even in the most challenging of circumstances."*
— *Laura (redesigningyourhealth.com)*

**Sources**
*Heal Your Headache: The 1-2-3 Program for Taking Charge of Your Pain* by David Buchholz, MD. Workman; 2002.
More Migraine-Free Cooking
(http://moremigrainefreecooking.blogspot.com/p/what-can-i-eat.html)

# *Ocular Migraines Facts*

*"It can be difficult for a doctor to make a diagnosis of vertigo caused by migraine. That's because people who have these headaches often have other conditions that may cause dizziness. This can include anxiety, depression, and positional low blood pressure."*
*— WebMD Medical Reference*

## What Are Ocular Migraines?
Ocular migraines cause vision loss or blindness lasting less than an hour, along with or following a migraine headache. Experts call these episodes *retinal*, *ophthalmic*, or *monocular* (meaning one eye) migraines.

## Warning Signs and Symptoms
Vision problems that affect one eye include:
- Flashing lights
- Blind spots in your field of vision
- Blindness in the eye

Vision loss can be a complication of retinal migraines. Headaches that last from four to 72 hours tend to:
- Affect one side of your head
- Feel moderately or very painful
- Pulsate in intensity

Feel worse when you're physically active Other symptoms include:
- Nausea
- Vomiting
- Unusual sensitivity to light or sound

An important symptom is when the vision loss only affects one eye.
A regular migraine with an aura, which can involve flashing lights and blind spots in the vision, is a common problem and affects about 20 percent of people who have migraines.

## Statistics
This problem is rare and affects about one in 200 people who have migraines.

# *Vertigo Facts*

## What is vertigo?
Vertigo is caused by issues with the inner ear — such as Benign Paroxysmal Positional Vertigo (or BPPV), which develops as tiny calcium particles build up in the ear canals; Meniere's disease, which is caused by fluid pressure in the ear; and Vestibular neuritis, a viral infection of the inner ear nerves.

All of these cause the body to become unbalanced and create a feeling that the world spinning, dizzy spells that come and go for about 20 seconds as your head changes positions.

## Warning Signs and Symptoms
- Distorted Balance
- Migraine Headaches
- Nausea
- Ringing in the Ears
- Fatigue
- Sweating
- Hearing Loss
- Twitching Eyes
- Ear Pressure
- Panic Attacks

## Statistics
90 million Americans suffer from vertigo, dizziness or balance problems. It is the second most common complaint heard in doctor's offices, and will occur in 70% of the nation's population at some time in their lives.

## Further Resources and Helpful Websites
National Eye Institute (www.nei.nih.gov)
WebMD (www.webmd.com)
Active Beat (www.activebeat.co)
Neuro Kinetics (www.neuro-kinetics.com)

# Part VII

# Bacterial Infections

*17*

# The Lifetime of Discovery
## of Natural Solutions to Illness

*"Take care of your body. It's the only place you have to live."*
*— Jim Rohn*

---

**Why Do People Get Sick?**
Donna's discovery of how natural solutions can keep people healthy and heal those who are sick began 25 years ago. It was after the birth of her second child, when she began to feel sick all the time for no apparent reason. She experienced joint pain, burning sensations, a constant low-grade fever while feeling cold, severe lymph pain, liver pain, and stomachache. And she felt terribly tired throughout the day.

During all of this, she learned that her father was diagnosed with bladder cancer. Plus, her children were also constantly sick. Her daughter suffered from nonstop ear infections. The antibiotics she took over and over again didn't seem to help. Her son had a chronic cough and was lucky enough to not notice the green phlegm that constantly drained from his nose. The four courses of antibiotics prescribed to him likewise didn't help.

All this made Donna wonder why people get sick. Being a registered nurse, she started her own investigation, and it was the beginning of her health-quest journey. That journey led her to discover the lifestyle that allowed her to stay healthy and feel vibrant and happy.

She sought the help of others, and it was a naturopath who suggested that she give up sugar and gluten. At this time, there was very little information on how sugar and gluten affect the body and influence our inflammation. So she tried it. Next, she gave up dairy. Her family did too.

It was a gradual process of healing, but her kids stopped getting sick and Donna's symptoms began to fade away. She still had stomach discomfort, but after introducing raw milk into her diet, the difficulty disappeared. Donna concluded that to fully recover, her body needed raw fat and probiotics that the raw milk provided. And after 10 years of sticking to her diet, she experience complete recovery.

Today, every naturopath is quick to provide information on dairy, sugar,

118

and gluten. Probiotics are also much more available. So Donna was a pioneer decades in front of the mainstream. She has been following the teachings of the Weston A. Price Foundation (www.westonaprice.org) for 15 years. She's a strong believer and committed raw foodie. And as a result, she hasn't been sick for 15 years.

## An Unfortunate Bite

In 2010, Donna was bitten by a tick between the toes on her left foot and contracted Lyme disease. Her foot began to turn black and a rash appeared over both of her legs. She felt severe fatigue.

Donna went to see a doctor and was prescribed antibiotics. *She refused taking the antibiotics, as she believed that she had an antibiotic resistance and didn't feel it would help. Instead, she followed her own line of treatment, which included four equally vital components.

1. BioMat — A state-of-the-art light technology that reverses degenerative disease cycles and speeds cellular renewal.
2. Biofeedback machine — A mind-body technique that teaches patients how to influence their autonomic nervous systems, the part of the body that controls involuntary physical functions such as blood pressure, heart rate, muscle tension, and brainwave frequency. This is done by attaching an electronic "cue" (usually a beep or visual image on a screen) to a measurable physiologic process. A person can thus monitor his or her internal responses and develop a sense of how to move them in positive ways.
3. Una De Gato (cat's claw) — An herb in the traditional medicine of Peru that has been used to treat numerous health conditions. Scientific research has revealed some of the active constituents and potential benefits including immune busting, anti-inflammatory, and cancer prevention.
4. High quality raw food diet with raw milk and absolutely no sugar or gluten.

In just three months, she felt better. In six months, she felt completely healed and back to normal. It's been over 25 years since Donna started her search for the root cause of each of her and her family members' health problems that led her to find real natural solutions, which do not cause any additional problems. She is one of those true pioneers who take a leap of faith to find the way and show the rest of us the path.

*"Through exploring nature, nurture, and nutrition, we find our true spiritual being."*

— *Donna (www.rawheal.com)*

# *Lime Disease Facts*

*"According to a new CDC estimate, more than 300,000 Americans are diagnosed with a tick-borne disease each year. The new number was presented at the 2013 International Conference on Lyme Borreliosis and Other Tick-Borne Diseases, being held in Boston."*
*— Harvard Health Publications, Harvard Medical School*

## What Is Lime Disease?
Lyme disease is caused by the bacterium *Borrelia burgdorferi* and is transmitted to humans through the bite of infected blacklegged ticks.

## Warning Signs and Symptoms
Lyme disease imitates a variety of illnesses, and its severity can vary. In the early stages of Lyme disease, one may experience flu-like symptoms:

- Stiff neck
- Chills
- Fever
- Swollen lymph nodes
- Headaches
- Fatigue
- Muscle aches
- Joint pain
- A large, expanding skin rash around the area of the tick bite

In more advanced stage of disease the symptoms may include:

- Erythma migrans, the telltale rash which occurs in about 70% to 80% of cases in the first few weeks.
- Arthritis.
- Neurological symptoms.
- Heart problems.
- Other symptoms including eye inflammation and severe fatigue.

## Statistics
In 2013, 95% of confirmed Lyme disease cases were reported from 14 states:

- Connecticut
- Delaware
- Maine

- Maryland
- Massachusetts
- Minnesota
- New Hampshire
- New Jersey
- New York
- Pennsylvania
- Rhode Island
- Vermont
- Virginia
- Wisconsin

**Further Resources and Helpful Websites**
Centers for Disease Control and Prevention (www.cdc.gov)
WebMD (www.webmd.com)

*\*Please note: This advice is not recommended for the general public. If you've been diagnosed with lime disease, you may need antibiotics. This was Donna's personal choice due to her having an antibiotic resistance.*

# Part VIII

# Adverse Drug Reactions

## 18
## Getting a Second Chance at Life And Gaining a New Outlook on One's Lifestyle

*"I don't understand why asking people to eat a well-balanced vegetarian diet is considered drastic, while it is medically conservative to cut people open and put them on cholesterol lowering drugs for the rest of their lives."*
*— Dean Ornish, MD*

Rudy comes from a large Italian family. He was raised on the heavy, rich foods his mother prepared, like lasagna, meatballs, and heavy cheese on everything. When his mother didn't cook, she ordered pizza for the family — usually with meat toppings. Rudy was the oldest of six children, and if he didn't eat quickly enough, someone else would eat his meal. So inhaling his food became a way of life.

Nine years ago, when Rudy decided to take his own family on a trip to New York over Christmas, everybody was excited about experiencing the city's famous Christmas magic and dining in Manhattan together.

On the second day of the trip, after a long day of walking, Rudy felt a massive muscle pain. It continued to worsen and the family had to drive him back to Massachusetts, so Rudy could crawl into bed. He ended up not being able to get out of his bed for the next six months.

When Rudy called his doctor, the doctor suggested that he stop taking a statin drug that Rudy had been prescribed to lower his cholesterol level. No further explanation was offered. When he pressed his doctor for more information, he couldn't get any answers. He called other doctors, and not one would openly admit that it was the statin drug that had caused his pain. And no one would make an official diagnosis that could explain Rudy's muscle damage.

Rudy's oldest daughter, Shayna, decided to do her own research on statins and learned a great deal about their side effects, like muscle weakness, pain, and muscle damage. She also learned that there were many people who were prescribed statin drugs and, as a result, struggled with similar issues.

Rudy was in constant pain, and his family was terrified. There were times they thought he was dying. Soon he wasn't able to run the family business, and Shayna, a first-year college student at the time, had to take over much of the day-to-day operation.

To help relieve his pain, Rudy was prescribed Vicodin, a powerful painkiller that's a combination opioid narcotic analgesic drug. As his pain grew, he took more, and soon became addicted to it. Finally, Rudy's doctor took him off Vicodin and prescribed him another strong medication designed to help drug addicts get clean.

During all of this, Rudy's blood pressure skyrocketed, so he was put on blood pressure medication. Every time he went to see a doctor he felt like he was put on a new medication and had to contend with new side effects. It became a vicious cycle.

The year he celebrated his 50$^{th}$ anniversary, Rudy was put on disability. He was still a young man, but all he could do was lie on the couch. He decided that he'd had enough. He wanted to be healthier and feel better, but his doctors didn't have the information he needed, and rarely had time for him. He realized that if he wanted to get better, it was up to him and no one else.

Rudy had suffered from high cholesterol for years. He also had frequent acid reflex and numerous digestive issues. He had a sense that this was related to his diet, but he couldn't get any guidance from his doctors. After years of wolfing down heavy, processed foods on the go, he decided that his first step to getting better would be to learn how to eat healthier.

**Eating Better, Living Better**
Rudy discovered that eating an anti-inflammatory diet and drinking lots of water helped keep his cholesterol at the normal level. Slowing down and eating mindfully helped keep his blood pressure down. Making better choices when choosing snacks — and not indulging on bread and pasta — has led to significant weight loss. He also takes supplements, including multivitamins, a B-complex, and vitamin D3.

Each improvement to his health encouraged him to do more. He began going to physical therapy, which helped him heal his muscle damage. He swims, which provides exercise that's not hard on his joints. Last year, on Shayna's birthday, after 30 years of smoking, Rudy gave up cigarettes.

He is also making himself feel better by reading motivational books, and he's taking steps to better deal with his seasonal affective disorder. New England's cold, long winters often left him feeling depressed. For a change, over the last couple of winters he's gone south, to Florida, and has been feeling much better.

Because Rudy grew up being the oldest son in a big family, he's used to everyone coming to him for help. And he loves helping people and is used to putting himself last. But now he realizes that if he takes better care of himself, he's better equipped to help others.

**Back on His Feet**
Today Rudy is feeling better than he did nine years ago. He's enthusiastic about life, feels good about his future, and has his spark back. He's also excited about everything that his children have going on in their lives and wants to be a part of it all.

He has more control over his body and is a lot more mindful than he's ever been. And he's not taking any narcotics or painkillers. He's walking again, with just a slight limp. After that Christmas vacation in New York, Rudy has made a lot of changes in his diet and lifestyle. He credits Shayna's determination with leading him on his journey. She helped him not give up on himself and become a better man.

With the help of others, Rudy made a powerful transformation from a stressed-out business owner who didn't take care of himself to a conscientious man who values and appreciates his health and well-being.

---

*"I never thought I would have a business based in health and wellness until my father became disabled from taking a statin drug to lower his cholesterol."*
*— Shayna (www.shaynamahoney.com)*

## *Statin Drugs and Their Side Effects Facts*

*"Statin side effects can be uncomfortable, making it seem like the risks outweigh
the benefits of these powerful cholesterol-lowering medications.
Consider the risks and benefits."*
— *Mayo Clinic*

**What Are Statins?**
Statins are a class of drugs often prescribed to help lower cholesterol
levels in the blood.

**What Are Statin Drugs Side Effects?**
According to WebMD, most people who take statin drugs tolerate them
very well. But some people experience side effects. The most common
statin side effects include:

- Headache
- Difficulty sleeping
- Flushing of the skin
- Muscle aches, tenderness, or weakness (myalgia)
- Drowsiness
- Dizziness
- Nausea or vomiting
- Abdominal cramping or pain
- Bloating or gas
- Diarrhea
- Constipation
- Rash

Statins also carry warnings that memory loss, mental confusion, high
blood sugar, and type 2 diabetes are possible side effects. They may also
interact with other medications you take.

**Which Statin Side Effects Are Serious?**
Statins are associated with a few rare, but potentially serious, side effects
including:

- Myositis, inflammation of the muscles.
- Rhabdomyolysis, extreme muscle inflammation and damage.

There are over 900 studies proving statins adverse effects. Statins deplete

127

your body of CoQ10 and if you take statin drugs without taking CoQ10, your health is at serious risk.

**Warning Signs and Symptoms**
If you experience any unexplained joint or muscle pain, tenderness, or weakness while taking statins, you should call your doctor immediately. The statin medications that are approved for use in the U.S. include:
- Lipitor
- Livalo
- Mevacor or Altocor
- Zocor
- Pravachol
- Lescol
- Crestor

**Statistics**
Since their arrival on the market, statins have been among the most prescribed drugs in the U.S. with about 17 million users. One in four Americans over the age of 45 are now taking a statin drug.

**Further Resources and Helpful Websites**
WebMD (http://www.webmd.com)

**Additional Reading**
http://articles.mercola.com/sites/articles/archive/2010/07/20/the-truth-about-statin-drugs-revealed.aspx
"The Great Cholesterol Myth: Why Lowering Your Cholesterol Won't Prevent Heart Disease — and the Statin-Free Plan That Will" by Stephen T. Sinatra, Jonny Bowden
"How Statin Drugs Really Lower Cholesterol: And Kill You One Cell at a Time" by James B. and Hannah Yoseph
"The Truth About Statins: Risks and Alternatives to Cholesterol-Lowering Drugs" by Barbara H. Roberts M.D.

# Part IX

# Environmental Diseases

## 19

## *The Missing Piece of the Healing Puzzle That Completes the Picture in Solving Your Health Problems*

*"We need to accept the seemingly obvious fact that a toxic environment can make people sick and that no amount of medical intervention can protect us."*
— *Andrew Weil*

---

Phyllis is a beautiful, active woman who exudes energy. She attributes her good health to her awareness of the impact that electricity and radio frequency have on our bodies. She learned about this while studying building biology, a field that complemented her interests in disease prevention. She has always understood the importance of good nutrition and a healthy life style. However, through building biology, she realized that external environmental factors also play an important role in our well-being.

Phyllis likes to say that while we can't always control our outdoor environment, we're fully in charge of our indoor environment.

### Good Sleep and Strong Immunity

When Phyllis acquired her own testing equipment to measure electromagnetic fields (EMF), including radio frequencies (RF), she began by testing her own house. After detecting that her cordless phone was emitting very strong RF waves — much higher than her cell phone Phyllis switched to a corded phone.

Next she measured electric and magnetic fields emanating from her home's electrical system. She detected strong electric fields near her bed. After determining which circuits were the cause, she turned them off.

The next morning, it took Phyllis a long time to wake up. It was almost as if she were emerging from a coma. She realized that she hadn't gotten up once during the night, which was rare for her. She typically experienced light, fitful sleep, but for the first time in a long time, she slept like a log.

Initially, Phyllis thought it might be a coincidence. But after a few more nights, her sound sleeping continued. People around her began to comment on her increased energy level. She felt better and was a lot more energetic.

## Chronic Pain and Invisible Solution

Years ago, Phyllis fell while horseback riding and has since experienced pain in her back. Since that accident, when she overexerts herself, the discomfort gets much worse. A couple years ago, Phyllis was shoveling snow and started to feel the familiar back pain setting in. She decided to take it easy for a week or so and let the pain subside. But her back didn't improve. Instead, the discomfort intensified, and Phyllis didn't understand why.

Phyllis discussed her back pain with friends while dining in a small restaurant. Suddenly, it occurred to her that maybe the reason for her difficulties had to do with the RF energy that she had been subjected to while traveling and doing her work. It was a cold night, and she and her friends were seated alone. She asked her friends to turn off their cell phones to see if she would feel any different. In about 10 minutes, one of them turned to Phyllis and asked how she was feeling. She realized that she was feeling much better. An hour later, though, a group of people came into the restaurant and the pain came back instantly. Surely, these people had their cellphones with them, she reasoned, and the phones were turned on. So Phyllis knew this was the reason why her pain came back.

This story proves how difficult it is for people to protect themselves from RF waves. You can't smell it or see it, so it's not easy to make the connection between the trigger and the physical symptoms. When Phyllis came home that evening, she decided to keep her cell phone off for a couple of days to see if the pain would go away completely. Sure enough, it did.

She now looks back on this accident as a gift because it was an eye-opener about how electromagnetic radiation can be the cause of a problem while being difficult to detect or measure.

## Heart Arrhythmia and Its Hidden Causes

Years before Phyllis got involved with building biology, she lived in a different house with her husband, a hard-core technology and gadget geek. They had wireless internet and cordless phones — and had recently upgraded to more powerful versions.

Soon after, Phyllis developed arrhythmia and ended up going to the hospital. She was premenopausal and assumed her symptoms were hormonal. However, now she knows that the reason for her arrhythmia was that she and her husband began using the all-new gadgets just prior to the accident. At the time, there was little understanding about the potential dangers lurking within technology.

Most people who contact Phyllis are experiencing symptoms they can't explain. Usually, they've already tried to get help from their doctors and either don't like the answers or don't want to undergo the treatment prescribed. So almost in all instances, this is about people whose symptoms were not adequately explained by medical professionals or the solutions they were offered seemed to be focused on minimizing the symptoms — not actually taking care of the problem.

There are a number of situations where the electromagnetic piece was not the main problem, but the trigger to expand the symptoms. For instance, Phyllis frequently deals with people who have suffered from mold exposure or have contracted Lyme disease. These conditions are linked in that they can both result from a compromised immune system — and the electromagnetic piece just aggravates it even further. Thus, by solving and reducing the electromagnetic fields around us, we can create a more nurturing environment to heal.

**Healthy Inside and Out**
As Phyllis continued to improve the EMF in her environment, she discovered that she was rarely getting sick. She was already generally healthy, but she still saw a startling improvement in her wellbeing and her ability to defend herself against day-to-day germs and all the other stuff that we're all exposed to.

She has been doing this work for six years, and her sleep improvements continue to this day. She also had many clients reporting to her that they couldn't believe the quality of their sleep after making simple changes in their houses.

We know that both quantity and quality of sleep influence the body's healing process and have an extraordinary impact on our quality of life. Thus, setting up the best conditions for sleep is vital for our wellbeing. And we sleep soundly when we're breathing healthy air and are protected from EMF, dirty electricity, and RF microwaves.

Phyllis admits that she's fortunate to have a home that is safe, whereas most people don't. Regrettably, most of us don't know what's going on in our homes and don't know who to go to in order to find out. Luckily, today the field of building biology is ever-growing.

*"I am dedicated to identifying root causes of disease and applying the science of environmental health to indoors building spaces as part of a total wellness program."*

*— Phyllis (www.yoursafeandsoundhome.com)*

# *Building Biology Facts*

*"Protecting the environment is everyone's responsibility, and starts with understanding the issues ... Learn what you can do to protect the environment in your home, workplace, and community."*
*— U.S. Environmental Protection Agency*

## What Is Building Biology?

Building biology is a field of building science investigating the indoor living environment for a variety of irritants. Practitioners believe the environment of residential, commercial and public buildings can affect the health of the occupants, producing a restful or stressful environment. Important areas of building biology:

- Building Materials and Processes
- Electromagnetic Fields (EMFs)
- Indoor Air Quality (IAQ)

Using sophisticated equipment, building biology specialists measure a variety of factors to gain a thorough understanding of a home environment. Their priorities are the most-occupied areas, such as sleeping areas, nurseries, and home offices.

## Statistics

Many health problems including eczema, cancer, and chronic fatigue syndrome have been linked to electromagnetic fields (EMF), dirty electricity, and RF microwave radiation. U.S. Environmental Protection Agency (EPA) cites indoor pollution as a "Top 5" health risk.

## Further Resources and Helpful Websites

U.S. Environmental Protection Agency (www.epa.gov)
The International Institute for Building Biology and Ecology (hbelc.org)
History of health effects from microwave technologies
(http://www.cellphonetaskforce.org/wp-content/uploads/2011/06/Electro
magneticHypersensitivity.pdf)
Smart Meters & Dangers from Other Similar RF Microwave Sources
(http://www.scribd.com/doc/99065792/Smart-Meter-Fact-Sheet)
Depth of Sleep and Health
(http://www.sleepfoundation.org/article/how-sleep-works/what-happens-
when-you-sleep)

Toxic Household Chemicals
(http://www.womensvoices.org/avoid-toxic-chemicals/)
Personal Care Product Safety Database
(http://www.ewg.org/skindeep/)
Tap Water Quality
(http://www.ewg.org/tap-water/home)
Medical society of environmental medicine
(http://aaemonline.org/)
Scientific views of EMF health risks
(http://electromagnetichealth.org/quotes-from-experts/)
World Health Organization Assessment of RF microwave dangers
(http://www.who.int/mediacentre/factsheets/fs193/en/index.html)
Actions to promote safe wireless
(http://citizensforsafetechnology.org/about-cst,1,0)

# *Part X*

# *Organ Transplant/Transplant Living*

THE POWER OF THE EDUCATED PATIENT

## A Mother's Choice: Give Up or Fight

*"God could not be everywhere, and therefore he made mothers."*
*— Rudyard Kipling*

---

All babies cry, but not all babies cry all the time. When Kian was born he seemed constantly irritated. He cried incessantly. It couldn't have been easy on him. It certainly wasn't easy on his mother, Nishma. When he was four weeks old, Nishma took him in for a scheduled checkup. After a quick examination, Kian was sent straight to the hospital. And then things got really challenging.

Kian was diagnosed with a liver disease. He spent a full week at the local hospital while doctors performed countless examinations and procedures. At the end of the week, Kian and Nishma were sent to a live-in hospital. As time went on, fear crept in. Especially when Nishma was told Kian may not survive. She spent days crying, nights praying — and all the while weighing the many choices and possible outcomes facing her and her family.

At just five weeks old, Kian wasn't gaining weight and wasn't growing. His doctors discovered that his gallbladder was completely blocked with bile. They removed it and reattached his intestines to his liver. At seven months, Kian was put on a waiting list for a liver transplant. Nishma was told that he wouldn't survive longer than six months without it. Luckily, two months later, they got a call that a liver was available, and Kian got a transplant.

### Living After a Lifesaving Operation
Kian was smiling two days after the operation. He finally began putting on weight. He was slightly slower to develop than some other babies — he started walking at 17 months — but he was a happy boy now. Nishma and her husband spent the next two years in and out of hospitals.

Any illness that Kian developed — even a simple cold — could rile up his immune system and cause it to attack his liver. Kian's doctors worked tirelessly to prevent his body from destroying his transplanted liver. It was a soul-breaking process, and Nishma knew that she had two choices: give up or fight. She chose to fight.

When Kian was in the hospital fighting for his life, Nishma stayed focused on taking care of whatever needed to be done. When she was finally able to take Kian home, she meticulously went over everything that happened. It was then that the gravity of their situation hit her, and a backlog of emotions worked its way out. She got depressed. She became anxious. She needed to find a new direction, so she researched alternatives.

Nishma learned how to help Kian nutritionally, emotionally, and spiritually. From his birth, Kian had taken so many antibiotics and other drugs that his whole system was messed up. Nishma started implementing alternative holistic methods to building up his immunity, and he became noticeably stronger.

**Today**
Today Kian is nine years old, strong, and enjoying fourth grade. He's roughly the same height and weight as the other kids in his class. If you met him and couldn't see the scar across his stomach, you'd have no idea that he'd undergone a liver transplant.

He's healthy overall and gets sick less often than his classmates. When he does fall ill, Nishma makes sure that he fully heals before sending him back to school. He continues to take his immune-suppressant drugs, and Nishma feeds him supplements to "bust up" his immune system so that he can fight infections. In the morning she gives him zinc, vitamin D3, vitamin C, and fish oil. In the evening, she feeds him probiotics. Nishma credits Kian's healthy gut with helping him fight off infection.

Because he's rarely sick, people often forget about his condition. However, he still needs to be careful when others around him are ill. When his schoolmates are sick with infection, Kian's teacher lets Nishma know. Nishma then takes precautions in building up Kian's immune system by giving him an extra dose of probiotics or vitamins.

**Embracing the Reality**
Kian has learned to appreciate the struggle that made him different, though it used to bother him quite a bit. He didn't understand why he had to be different than the other kids, why he was the only one with a scar across his stomach.

When Kian was five years old, his parents took him to the Transplant Games, in London. At the games, all the participating kids lifted their tops

139

up and Kian was astonished, telling his mom, "Wow. I'm not the only one!" Since that day, he embraces what makes him different. What makes him special.

Last year, Kian took part in the American Transplant Games for the first time. He earned two gold medals and a silver. He's preparing to represent the United States for the World Championships next year.

Nishma says that what she and her husband went through with Kian taught them how precious each day is. That it could be taken away tomorrow. Each day she and her husband fight to keep Kian healthy and alive. But she's happy they're doing it together, adding, "What parent in this position wouldn't do the same thing and choose to fight?"

---

*"I believe that every child has a right to a long, healthy life. I believe that simple changes can make extensive improvements."*

— *Nishma (www.essentialharmony.net)*

# *Liver Transplant Facts*

*"The first human whole organ transplant 60 years ago — a living kidney transplant — changed the landscape of the medical world. Since then, transplants of skin, kidneys, hearts, lungs, corneas, and livers have become commonplace but due to a shortage of donor organs, more than 120,000 patients are still on waitlists for organ transplantation in the United States alone."*
*— National Institutes of Health (NIH)*

## What Is a Liver Transplant?
A liver transplant is a surgical procedure to remove a diseased liver and replace it with a healthy liver from a donor. Most liver transplant operations use livers from deceased donors, though a liver may also come from a living donor. The liver performs many complex functions in the body:

- Makes most proteins needed by the body
- Metabolizes, or breaks down, nutrients from food to make energy
- Prevents shortages of nutrients by storing certain vitamins, minerals, and sugar
- Makes bile, a compound needed to digest fat and absorb vitamins A, D, E, and K
- Makes most of the substances that regulate blood clotting
- Helps the body fight infection by removing bacteria from the blood
- Removes potentially toxic by-products of certain medications

## Warning Signs and Symptoms of Liver Disease
Patients with mild liver disease may have few or no symptoms or signs. Patients with more serious liver disease develop symptoms and signs that may be nonspecific or specific. Nonspecific symptoms include:

- Fatigue
- Weakness
- Vague abdominal pain

Loss of appetite Specific symptoms include:

- Yellowing of the skin (jaundice) due to the accumulation of bilirubin in the blood
- Itching
- Easy bruising due to decreased production of blood clotting factors by the diseased liver

Severe, advanced liver disease with cirrhosis symptoms include:
- Fluid accumulation in the legs (edema) and abdomen (ascites)
- Mental confusion or coma
- Kidney failure
- Vulnerability to bacterial infections
- Gastrointestinal bleeding

**When Is a Liver Transplant Needed?**

A liver transplant is considered when the liver no longer functions adequately (liver failure). The following conditions may result in chronic liver failure:
- Chronic hepatitis with cirrhosis
- Primary biliary cirrhosis (a rare condition where the immune system inappropriately attacks and destroys the bile ducts)
- Sclerosing cholangitis (scarring and narrowing of the bile ducts inside and outside of the liver, causing the backup of bile in the liver)
- Biliary atresia (a rare disease of the liver that affects newborns)
- Alcoholism
- Wilson's disease (a rare inherited disease with abnormal levels of copper throughout the body, including the liver)
- Hemochromatosis (a common inherited disease where the body has too much iron)
- Alpha-1 antitrypsin deficiency (an abnormal buildup of alpha-1 antitrypsin protein in the liver, resulting in cirrhosis)
- Liver cancer

Liver failure has many causes, including:
- Liver cirrhosis
- Biliary duct atresia
- Cystic fibrosis
- Early-stage liver cancer
- Hemochromatosis
- Primary biliary cirrhosis
- Primary sclerosing cholangitis
- Wilson's disease

**Risks**

Liver transplant surgery carries a risk of significant complications, including:

- Bile duct complications, including bile duct leaks or shrinking of the bile ducts
- Bleeding
- Blood clots
- Failure of donated liver
- Infection
- Memory and thinking problems
- Rejection of donated liver

**Side Effects of Antirejection Medications**
After a liver transplant you'll take medications for the rest of your life to help prevent your body from rejecting the donated liver. These medications can cause a variety of side effects, including:
- Bone thinning
- Diabetes
- Diarrhea
- Headaches
- High blood pressure
- High cholesterol

**Statistics**
Six-thousand liver transplants are performed annually in the U.S., and the number continues to rise.

**Further Resources and Helpful Websites**
American Liver Foundation (www.liverfoundation.org)

# Part XI

## Unknown/Undiagnosed Mystery Disorders

## 21
## *A Key Ingredient to Good Health —*
## *the Inner Power to Heal*

*By Janet Verney*

*"Every struggle in your life has shaped you into the person you are today. Be thankful for the hard times; they have made you stronger."*
*— Unknown*

---

Have you ever lost something and felt like you'll go nuts until you find it? Well, that's what happened to Janet some thirty years ago. Only it wasn't an object that she lost, but her health.

Dialing back to her early twenties, she's living in an apartment in Hartford, CT. One beautiful, sunny morning she decides to go for a run. As she starts, her chest is heavy and, with each step she takes, it gets harder and harder to breathe. She tries to ignore it and hopes the feeling will go away, but it keeps getting worse. She begins obsessing about what's wrong and why this is happening to her; at the same time, she feels a bit of panic bubbling up in her chest from not being able to take a full, deep breath.

Later in the day, she heads to the doctor, who diagnoses her with a bad case of bronchitis. At least that's what he thinks it is. He prescribes an antibiotic, which seems to help a little, yet the congestion is still there. In fact, it never goes away.

This health crisis is suddenly front and center in Janet's life. She goes to doctor after doctor, and each one has a diagnosis that is subsequently disproven by another. She feels discouraged and, with each infection, more and more afraid of what's to come.

Janet's primary care physician (PCP) insists the problem is asthma, and proceeds to prescribe a multitude of meds. She takes them faithfully, even though it doesn't feel right. (You know that feeling down deep in your gut when something just isn't right.) In the long run, the medicines make her feel worse. The prednisone has her all hyped up, the albuterol makes her feel jittery, and the theophylline makes her feel lightheaded and shaky on her feet. That's when she begins seeing a pulmonologist. After several breathing tests, he rules out asthma, Janet takes herself off the meds, and shortly thereafter she finds a new PCP.

The infections get worse and more frequent, and are greatly interfering with Janet's day-to-day work and play. She never knows when she's going to have a bad day, so it's hard to plan ahead. She ends up canceling events (a date with a friend, an outing to some place fun) or calling in sick to work. She loves public speaking, yet she is embarrassed by her cough. She is often asked if it is a smoker's cough, and then she goes into her spiel about having an undiagnosed cough.

When she explains that we don't know what it is, she senses judgment in the questioner's eyes and self-doubt creeps in; she feels like one of the "misfit toys." By now, she has been told by a few doctors that maybe it's all in her head. More self-doubt, some sadness, and a big dose of self-pity add up to a feeling of depression.

Her lungs were filled with a sticky white fluid, causing chronic infections; she was not properly digesting protein and fats, and became nutrient deficient. Janet kept thinking, it will come back, she'll get better, especially when they (the doctors) figure out what it is and how best to treat it. Well, they always have the answers, a bit of advice, a pill to give, a few stitches to make her good as new.

But this time it was different.

Janet was passed from doctor to doctor and each one had a different idea about what it could be. One test after another, and they kept coming back negative. In 2009 Janet was one of 100 patients in the country accepted to the National Institutes of Health's (NIH) Undiagnosed Disease Program. She spent a week at the NIH hospital campus undergoing a series of tests, interviews, and exams. She had a team of about fifty doctors studying her case.

It is very much like the famed TV show *House,* only a lot less dramatic and often without the diagnosis, which is how it was in Janet's case. Janet thinks that the hardest thing of all is the internal blame that creeps up all too often. That little voice whispers, "If you only did this, or that, you would get better." Too much time is spent on over thinking "what could this be."

Then there is the forever hopeful mode that there's a miracle cure out there, and with each new supplement or treatment, she would think "This is it, this will fix it," only to be disappointed once again.

The tests and procedures, and then hearing the results, took a toll on Janet but the worst was the negative chatter in her own mind that played over and over again like a bad rerun on TV or a song that you can't get out of your head. She would get so caught up in fear that she'd feel paralyzed — and withdraw from life. This type of thinking put Janet in a dark place and further eroded her overall health.

After many years of trying to find the diagnosis, Janet realized that her efforts would be better served by focusing on getting to the root of what caused this disease, to weed out the obstacles that were in her way to healing, and to fully nourish herself, inside and out. Shifting her attitude has been a key ingredient to living well, one day at a time.

Janet spent time at a healing institute, where she gained tremendous knowledge about the way food and lifestyle choices play key roles in our health (or lack thereof). She learned we can change our biology by the food choices we make. Through the exploration of food and nutrition, key ingredients became a primary path for her healing. Her passion for food and nutrition grew every day as she saw the difference food can make in the healing process.

As Janet learned about how toxic foods affect us and cause an imbalance in our bodies, she also discovered the hidden health risks of many of the products we put on our skin, and the chemicals we use to clean our homes. She learned to clean up not only her diet, but also the environment around her.

This was just the beginning of Janet's journey to find the healing strategies that helped her to live in wellness. She focused on unearthing the root cause, weeding out the obstacles in her way to healing, and nourishing her roots through a variety of practices, which are outlined in her book *ROOTS2Wellness*. She now thrives in health and happiness.

Janet knows she has this disease for a greater purpose in life, and she believes it is to help others to find *their* route to wellness. The life we are given is a gift, and when we bless the good and acknowledge the message from our challenges, we generate a flow of positive energy that envelops us in love, which is the ultimate cure.

---

*"As you set out on this healing journey, create your own road map to follow. Be prepared for detours, but having a route to follow will help you to stay on course."*

— *Janet (www.roots2wellness.com)*

# *Rare Disease or Orphan Disease Facts*

*"Trying to find an underlying diagnosis for many conditions can be a very long and frustrating experience. With more rare conditions, a diagnosis can often take many years."*
*— The National Organization for Rare Disorders (NORD)*
*the National Institutes of Health (NIH)*

## What Is a Rare Disease or Orphan Disease?
A rare disease, also referred to as an orphan disease, is any disease that affects a small percentage of the population. Most rare diseases are genetic, and are present throughout the person's entire life, even if symptoms do not immediately appear.

## Warning Signs and Symptoms
Symptoms of some rare diseases may appear at birth or in childhood, whereas others only appear once adulthood is reached.

## Statistics
According to the Office of Rare Diseases Research:
- There are approximately 7,000 different types of rare diseases and disorders, with more being discovered each day.
- 30 million people in the United States are living with rare diseases. This equates to 1 in 10 Americans, or 10% of the U.S. population.
- Similar to the United States, Europe has approximately 30 million people living with rare diseases.
- It is estimated that 350 million people worldwide suffer from rare diseases.
- 80% of rare diseases are genetic in origin, and thus are present throughout a person's life, even if symptoms do not immediately appear.
- Approximately 50% of the people affected by rare diseases are children.
- 30% of children with rare disease will not live to see their fifth birthday.
- Rare diseases are responsible for 35% of deaths in the first year of life.
- The prevalence distribution of rare diseases is skewed — 80% of

all rare disease patients are affected by approximately 350 rare diseases.

- According to the Kakkis EveryLife Foundation, 95% of rare diseases have not one single FDA approved drug treatment.
- During the first 25 years of the Orphan Drug Act (passed in 1983), only 326 new drugs were approved by the FDA and brought to market for all rare disease patients combined.
- According to the National Institutes of Health Office of Rare Disease Research, approximately 6% of the inquiries made to the Genetic and Rare Disease Information Center are in reference to an undiagnosed disease.
- Approximately 50% of rare diseases do not have a disease specific foundation supporting or researching their rare disease.

**Further Resources and Helpful Websites**
Genetic and Rare Diseases Information Center (rarediseases.info.nih.gov)
Global Genes - Allies in Rare Disease (globalgenes.org)

# *Afterword*

You have read the healing stories.
You have learned new strategies and approaches.
You have become an even more educated and empowered patient.
And as an empowered patient, you are your own best health advocate!

Use this power of knowledge to choose what would work best for you
from both — Alternative and Conventional Medicine.
These choices will set you off on your road to recovery and take you all
the way to your most vibrant health.

The German philosopher, Arthur Schopenhauer wrote:

*"All truth passes through three stages.
First, it is ridiculed.
Second, it is violently opposed.
Third, it is accepted as being self- evident."*

Today, some of us may feel that alternative medicine is a fraud.
Many may resist it.
And every day more and more of us recognize it as real and powerful.

Start from where you are.

Take what you are ready for and willing to.
Implement what you find helpful and explore what you consider worth
looking into.

This is your life and your health. Own it!

# Final Word
## (Thank You and Special Invitation)

*"Trust your instincts. It is your health and your life. Persist in finding
the care your deserve. Don't settle for less."*
— Kenneth R. Blanchard, PH.D., M.D.

---

We all become patients at some point in our lives. We may be sick and need help getting better. We might go in for a 'well' appointment, like an annual physical exam. Whatever the case, we all deserve the best healthcare there is — healthcare that not only helps us overcome our diseases but also enables us to get and stay strong and healthy.

Our storytellers have given you their proven strategies and shared the fundamental principles that guided them to recovery. They've empowered you by illuminating the path they took, so you can apply what they learned to your own health and well-being.

Everyone who shared their story with you is on *a mission to inspire, educate and empower more people*. However, we can only achieve it with *your help*. Encourage your friends, relatives, loved ones, clients, and patients to read, absorb, and apply the approaches used by our storytellers.

We want to stay in touch with you and support *you* in achieving *your most vibrant health and joyful life*. We also would love you to share your success stories with us. You can inspire more people, as well as read about others, at www.ThePowerOfTheEducatedPatient.com. On this website, you'll find "The Bottom-Line of Identifying Your Best HealthCare" quiz that will help you determine how educated and empowered you are as a patient. Additionally, we'll invite you for free to future seminars taught by health professionals and victorious conquerors over their diseases.

We would be honored to have the chance to learn about and from YOU! We look forward to meeting and greeting YOU!

For more strategies, insights, and information, email
**ThePowerOfTheEducatedPatient@gmail.com** or visit
**www.IreneHealthAndWellnessEducator.com**
**www.ThePowerOfTheEducatedPatient.com**
**https://www.facebook.com/ThePowerOfTheEducatedPatient**

# *About the Author*

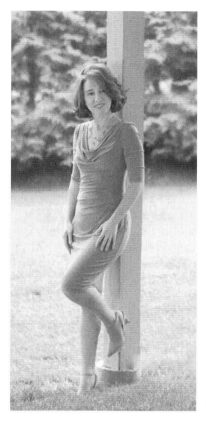

Irene Drabkin CHHC, AADP is a health and wellness educator and a speaker.

Irene is known for offering attention-grabbing highly effective seminars, retreats and private coaching programs on a variety of nutrition and lifestyle topics that help people manage stress, improve energy, overcome emotional eating and lose weight without constant dieting and deprivation.

Irene is a Transformational Wellness Expert and a Board Certified Integrative Nutrition Counselor accredited by Columbia University Teacher's College and the American Association of Drugless Practitioners.

Irene is a woman on a mission, who has dedicated her life to helping others listen to the wisdom of their bodies and to make lifestyle and food choices their greatest ally in reaching optimal health.

If you would like to invite Irene to speak to your group or organization, or find more information about her seminars, health and wellness coaching programs, please email **ThePowerOf TheEducatedPatient@gmail.com** or visit **www.IreneHealthAndWellnessEducator.com**

155

Every single conqueror of their disease shared the same three crucial requirements for healing and vibrant health:
- **Healthy lifestyle**
- **Wholesome diet and clean environment**
- **Emotional balance and spiritual health equilibrium**

***Here is the wisdom of confirmation from the experts:***

**Healthy Lifestyle**
"Your genetics load the gun. Your lifestyle pulls the trigger."

— Mehmet Oz, M.D.

Everyone has their own definition of a healthy lifestyle, and mine has come to mean making health a priority but not an obsession."

— Daphne Oz

"As I see it, every day you do one of two things: build health or produce disease in yourself."

— Adelle Davis

**Wholesome Diet and Clean Environment**
"We are all making life-or-death decisions every single day in terms of what we choose to put into our bodies and how we choose to use them."

— David Katz, M.D.

"The food you eat can be either the safest and most powerful form of medicine or the slowest form of poison."

— Ann Wigmore

"Today, more than 95% of all chronic disease is caused by food choice, toxic food ingredients, nutritional deficiencies and lack of physical exercise."

— Mike Adams

**Emotional Balance and Spiritual Health Equilibrium**
"Forgive yourself and others, live with hope, faith and love and watch the results in your life and in the lives you touch. Remember that success and healing refer to what you do with your life, not to how long you avoid death."

— Bernie Siegel, M.D.

"The more I observed human behavior, the more convinced I became that the key to health is understanding each person's individual needs, rather than following a set of predetermined rules. I saw plenty of evidence that having happy relationships, a fulfilling career, an exercise routine and a spiritual practice are even more important to health than a daily diet."

— Joshua Rosenthal

"You are not a mistake. You are not a problem to be solved. But you won't discover this until you are willing to stop banging your head against the wall of shaming and caging and fearing yourself."

— Geneen Roth

Printed in Great Britain
by Amazon.co.uk, Ltd.,
Marston Gate.